Hearing Loss Tips

For Those Who Have it, and Those Who Don't

By Linnaea Mallette

ABOUT THE COVER

The cover illustrates a hearing-impaired cat adjusting the volume of the hearing aids to hear the squeak of a mouse. A very meaningful sound for a cat, indeed!

There are millions of people who are missing the meaningful sounds of their life because of a hearing loss.

Cover design and book formatting by Circe Denyer

Images (non-photographic) GraphicsFactory.com

Edited by Sunil Suresh, Elance.com

Hearing test and equipment photographs by Circe Denyer

Childhood photo taken by Loyal Lewis (Linnaea's Dad)

Photograph of Bruce Mallette, courtesy of MalletteStringQuartet.com by Circe Denyer

Hearing aid images courtesy Oticon, used by permission

ISBN-13: 978-1495391330

ISBN-1495391337

I dedicate this book to all
who struggle with hearing loss.

I wish for you, connection.

Note: For your convenience and ease....important
charts and images used are available at
http://hearinglosstips.com/downloads.

Reference links for each chapter are located at the
end of each chapter.

ACKNOWLEDGEMENTS

To my husband, Bruce Mallette for his painstaking research on closed captioning, making watching movies more enjoyable and interesting
http://mallettestringquartet.com

To business partner and friend, Circe Denyer, for photographs, editing, book formatting and images
http://for17seconds.com

To Patrice Rifkind, Au.D., CCC-A,
Doctor of Audiology, Audiology Associates
for the technical edits and contributions
http://www.audiologyassociates.net

Toastmasters International, for my confidence
http://toastmasters.org

Table of Contents

PREFACE
BARBARA MASSEY

So much of what Linnaea writes is exactly what a lot of us have been thinking. We've also been thinking perhaps we are the only ones having this difficulty. It may sound harsh….but it's nice to know we're not alone.

It's funny that when our eyesight starts to diminish, we rush down to the store and get some of those little 'cheaters' or magnifying glasses; but when our hearing becomes a problem, we fight it tooth and nail. For years, we say 'uh?' and 'what?' Or as Linnaea points out…pretend we heard what was said. We laugh, nod, and hope the person has not just told us that someone we love died!

I gave a copy of Linnaea's book to my audiologist. I know even she could learn something that would be helpful to her and her patients

Linnaea presents so much important information within the covers of her book; it's impossible for me to single out a phrase or two that would appropriately tell you how much I enjoyed and learned from reading it. From 'Dangers' to 'Myths' to 'How hearing aids aren't the implements for perfectly restored hearing' (like I hoped they'd be). I love the chapter 'Benefits of Hearing Loss.' Wow, I didn't know there were ANY…until I read that chapter. Linnaea's insight helps make lemonade out of lemons, with a smile.

In short, the book is wonderful. It is as the cover promises: This book truly is:

INFORMATIVE!

HONEST!

FUNNY! And

INSPIRATIONAL!

I am proud to claim Linnaea not only an inspirational and great speaker and writer, but also a good friend.

Sincerely, Barbara J. Massey

INTRODUCTION

A lovely hygienist who had been cleaning my teeth for several years inspired the work I have compiled in this book. One day, after cleaning my teeth, she pulled down her facemask so I could read her lips and asked in her strong Russian accent, "Linnaea, my husband and I have noticed we are losing some of our hearing as we grow older. Any tips for us?"

I, taken by surprise – first by her question – then by the realization that I literally had a lifetime of experience on this topic – realized that my experience could be beneficial to those unfamiliar with the challenges of having, or interacting with, a person with a hearing loss.

I shared with her some of what I discuss in this book:

The three biggest myths associated with hearing loss

Three things she can ask of individuals to help her be part of the conversation

The dynamics of hearing that everyone uses and can be capitalized on when it comes to hearing loss

Some of the dangers of having a hearing loss

Some of the benefits of having a hearing loss

I could tell by her response that what I shared was tremendously helpful. She could relate to what I was sharing with what she and her husband had already been experiencing. She was deeply appreciative of my honesty and the survival tips I provided. I felt immensely satisfied because I knew if she fully embraced and practiced what I gave her, she and her husband could go on living full, active and satisfying lives despite their diminishing hearing.

That is when I realized it was time for me to share my insights, experiences and tips with a broader audience. I do so, not from an academic "schooled" point of view, although I certainly do draw upon some of those resources in this book, but, as a person who has struggled with this physical disability since early childhood. My sharing is honest – personal – from the gut, no-holds-barred. It has to be that way to be truly helpful.

Why?

Because the biggest challenge in my life was not the inability to hear well. It was the unwillingness to recognize the severity of the loss and, therefore, not seek the type of information and help that I share in this book.

So here it is. Hearing Loss Tips – For Those Who Have it and Those That Don't.

CHAPTER 1
WHY SHOULD YOU CARE ABOUT HEARING LOSS?

"The thing about hearing loss is that no one can see it. You simply can't look at a person and tell if they have a loss. Most people are so impatient and they just assume that the person with hearing loss is being rude, slow-witted" – Marion Ross (from Happy Days reflecting about the experiences of her hearing-impaired friend).

Have you ever interacted with a person with imperfect hearing? Chances are you have and did not know it; (we are professional bluffers). According to the National Institute on Deafness and Other Communication Disorders nearly 17 percent (36 million) American adults struggle with imperfect hearing.

You should care because hearing loss affects one's ability to communicate. According to a new Johns Hopkins', study, almost a fifth of Americans over 12 years old have difficulty communicating due to not being able to hear well.

The ability to communicate and stay connected has a direct effect on one's level of happiness, one's self esteem and quality of life. It may be a family member, friend, customer, client, employer, employee...or even you. ALL impacted by hearing loss.

This book focuses on those who have partial hearing loss – not those who are completely deaf and must rely on sign language to communicate. Partial loss is a tough place to be – in-between two worlds – not quite hearing impaired enough to be fully integrated into the deaf community – but not fully fitting in to the hearing world either.

This book seeks to help make that middle place easier to live in.

Chapter 1 References and Resources:

Dybala, P. (n.d).. *Happy Days Marion Ross*. Retrieved December 2014, from

Oncology Online:
http://www.audiologyonline.com/interviews/interview-with-marion-ross-mrs-1522

Johns Hopkins. (2011, November 14). *One in Five Americans Has a Hearing Loss*. Retrieved December 2013, from Johns Hopkins Medicine - News and Publications:
http://www.hopkinsmedicine.org/news/media/releases/one_in_five_americans_has_hearing_loss

CHAPTER 2:
MY STORY

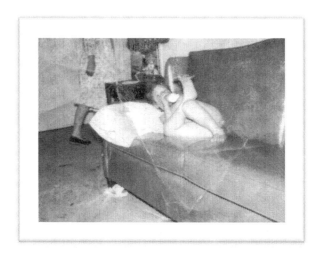

I joined the largest minority group – the physically disabled – when I was just four years old. I remember the point of entry. I was lying on a brown Naugahyde sofa, hot, kicking the covers off me. I do not know which of the three childhood diseases I had at that time – but I had a run of mumps, measles and chicken pox very close to one another. My brother, 7 years older, kept pulling the covers back over me. My mom was kneeling down next to me, one hand on my forehead, the other holding the mercury thermometer. I felt her hand tremble as she exclaimed with alarm, "Your sister has a fever of 106 degrees!"

It was then that I lost a significant amount of my hearing.

I can vividly recall when I realized I was different from my peers. I was at a friend's birthday party, sitting at a table surrounded by a bunch of kids my age. I recall the huge balloons that hung all around. I think they were the size of me. I recall this very sick feeling in my stomach that something was amiss. I just didn't feel connected to the party. I recall thinking "I am different. I don't fit." It was a very surreal feeling.

A few months later, sitting in our car waiting for dad to return from the hardware store, my mom asked me to listen to the ticking of my dad's wristwatch. I could not hear it. She held it up to the other ear. Still no sound. A subsequent visit to Children's Hospital confirmed my mom's fear… that 106-degree fever had seared off about 70% of my hearing. I will never forget the look on her face.

My mom was an alcoholic. I didn't want to be the reason she drank. So I decided, at a very young age, not to have my hearing loss be a problem – for anyone. That decision stuck with me for over 40 years, denying the extent of my loss. I did not educate myself about it. I did not seek much help. I lost out because of it.

I did attend a public elementary school from third grade on that had a special program for the deaf and the hard of hearing. I found the curriculum too slow and by seventh grade, I switched to a "normal" public school. I'm not sure it was the right decision in the long term. I suffered intense teasing in High School, so much so I dropped out one full semester in the 10th grade, and then dropped out entirely half way through the 12th grade. I learned just a few years ago that many of those "special needs" students I left behind received a college education, compliments of the State of California. I never went to college. I did not have parents who were aggressive in making sure I received support for what I needed. They trusted my bull-headed stubbornness and insistence that I didn't need special attention.

But, I did.

Not only for my hearing loss, but also for my self-esteem – which was dangerously low.

I once read that one of the characteristics of a person with a physical disability is the drive to prove oneself. When I was 23, I decided to do what could be considered improbable for one with a hearing loss — in order to be accepted, I started taking on challenges I really had no business taking on.

One of these was parachuting without a tandem partner (I don't think tandem jumping was an option in 1978)

I decided to try skydiving at Skyworld ™ at Lake Elsinore, California. I did not tell the instructors I had a hearing loss – although if they had been even slightly educated they might have picked up that I did have diminished hearing. If they did, I am surprised they let me jump unassisted.

I went through several hours of training on how to land without breaking my legs, and when to open the spare parachute. The winds were high when the training was finished so we had to wait several hours before we climbed aboard the big plane that took us up 1,800 feet so we could jump.

I jumped, attached to a ripcord, so the chute automatically opened after free falling for five seconds.

As I was floating down to the ground, the walkie-talkie strapped to my waist chattered at me. No way could I understand anything being said! I wondered if they were giving me any warnings. I wondered if I was floating to the ground too fast…and thought that maybe, I SHOULD open my spare chute. I frantically looked at the other parachutes around me; it seemed we were all going at about the same speed. But I wasn't absolutely sure.

Not wanting to appear stupid by opening my spare chute when it was not necessary, and therefore revealing I was half-deaf and couldn't hear what the walkie-talkie was instructing me to do… I did not open my spare chute. In looking back, I realize I chose DEATH over letting people know I was hearing impaired. That is how low my self-esteem was.

Obviously, I lived to tell the story. I jumped two more times after that first jump. Not so much because I loved doing it, but because I wanted to prove to myself and my friends that my hearing loss wasn't going to stop me from doing things "normal" people do and without assistance.

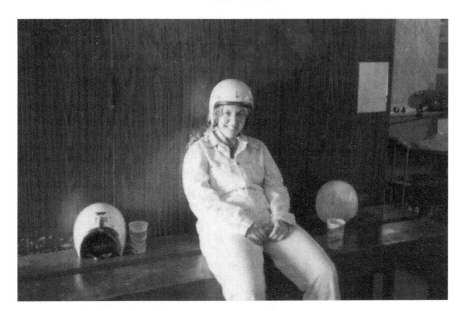

FIRST PARACHUTE JUMP CERTIFICATE

This Is To Certify That _____Linnaea P. Lewis_____ Successfully Completed

A Static Line Parachute Jump From An Aircraft In Flight

At Skyworld™, Lake Elsinore, California, A Parachutes Incorporated Center

On The __2__ Day Of __Sept__ In The Year __1978__

Jacques André Istel
President, Parachutes Incorporated
United States Instructor Certificate No. 1

Instructor 03520

Pretty risky business, wouldn't you say? That risky business of mine followed me into the workplace too.

In 1980, I joined the Office of Research Administration at UCLA and slowly worked my way up from an assistant to a Grant Officer. The position required extensive phone interactions – negotiating terms and conditions with Government, non-profit and industrial sponsors of research. It required an eye for detail. It also required good mathematical skills to analyze budgets (for which I am truly disabled). I took pride in having achieved the Grant Officer position with no college education, working amongst peers who were highly educated, many of them attorneys. However, I was also MISERABLE. And absent – a lot.

It all came crashing down in 1998, three years after I volunteered to be a "team leader" in ill-planned and ill-fated office reorganization. I was a dismal failure. The office wanted to dismiss me.

Having been in that organization for so long, I had a huge "database" of vocabulary unconsciously stored away that made speech comprehension easier (more on this in the Dynamics of Hearing Chapter). Seeking employment in an unfamiliar environment where sounds and words and people were all new while my confidence was at an all-time low, was not an option.

Consequently, I opted to take a huge demotion in position and pay while I sought to restore my confidence through the help of a therapist. This was all part of the worst three years of my life, and the inspiration for my first book about facing and overcoming adversity. The therapist helped me see that a big reason why I failed was that I simply was not in touch with my physical disability and the extent to which it affected my life.

It is a known fact that employees with disabilities are valuable assets. DuPont conducted a study of its employees with disabilities and in 1973 concluded that those employees with disabilities equal or exceed their able-bodied co-workers in allegiance, attendance and performance. It wasn't my disability that hurt my performance; it was that I did not acknowledge my limitations within the disability. It took that incredibly patient therapist to convince me of that fact. When she finally did, the first triumphant step I took was to change my voice mail to say, "Please speak slowly and enunciate numbers, you are leaving a message for a hearing-impaired person." The focus of my life from that point on shifted from proving me to others (so I would be accepted), to me being more accepting of my hearing loss and myself.

These experiences speak profoundly of the impact hearing loss can have on one's self esteem. My hearing loss, which contributed to my low self-esteem, prevented me from asking for assistance and even taking action to save my career and, as in the parachuting experience, my limbs and life.

In conclusion:

Hearing loss can affect one's self-esteem. Low self-esteem can cause one to take unhealthy risks. It is critical for parents of a child with a hearing disability to educate themselves, and their child, about all aspects of the disability early on, so he or she can live a full life with as little struggle as possible.

Chapter 2 References and Resources:

Linnaea Mallette's Book, "Read My Lips Tips for Success" http://www.linnaeamallette.com/books-by-linnaea-mallette/

Note: This book is being edited and updated for re-release in 2015 under the title of "Tips to Get Out of the Pits"

Berger, J. T. (n.d).. *Disabled Workers: Diamonds in the Rough*. Office Solutions Magazine.

Oshkosh Area Workforce Development Center. (n.d).. *Consumer Services / Disability Resources*. Retrieved October 17, 2014, from Oshkosh Area Workforce Development Center: http://www.oshkoshwdc.com/data/Studies_Related_to_the_Employment_of_Individuals_with_Disabilities.pdf

CHAPTER 3:
HOW WE HEAR

"...Seeing, hearing, feeling, are miracles, and each part and tag of me is a miracle..." – Walt Whitman

In order to understand hearing loss, it is important to have some idea of how we hear. Here is a very simple explanation:

Unlike our sense of vision, taste and smell, which are chemical reactions; our hearing is based on movement. Vibrations and physical movement. When something makes a noise, it sends vibrations, or sound waves, through the air. Our ears pick up these sounds and convert them into a form our brain can understand.

There are three parts to our ears — the outer ear, the middle ear and the inner ear.

Anatomy of the Ear

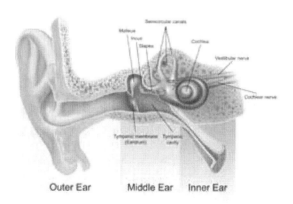

Outer Ear   Middle Ear   Inner Ear

Sound enters the ear through the ear canal and starts a vibration of the eardrum. The vibration is then transferred to the three bones of the middle ear — the hammer, the anvil, and finally the stirrup.

The stirrup passes those vibrations along a coiled tube shaped like a snail's shell in the inner ear called the cochlea.

Inside the cochlea, thousands of auditory hair cells transform the sound into electrical signals transmitted to the brain via the auditory nerve. Our brain deciphers all this and tells us what we are hearing.

In conclusion:

Our ears are sensitive, miraculous organs that give us our sense of hearing. However, people can develop hearing loss either due to natural causes or due to accidents. The next chapter describes the different types of hearing loss.

Chapter 3 References and Resources:

How We Hear
https://science.education.nih.gov/supplements/nih3/hearing/guide/info-hearing.htm

CHAPTER 4:
TYPES OF HEARING LOSS

"Sound is not only a guide to the practicalities of living....it is also an aesthetic pleasure." – G.C. Lichtenberg (Farewell to Fear)

According to the World Health Organization, hearing loss is defined as not being able to hear sounds of 20 decibels or less in the frequencies where the components of speech reside. Speech sounds begin at about 20 decibels for the "soft" consonants (f, s, th) and around 70 for the vowels (a, e, i, o, u).

There are two basic types of hearing loss — sensorineural and conductive. A person can have one or both types of losses in one or both of their ears. The types are classified by which part of the ear is damaged.

Sensorineural Hearing Loss (SNHL)

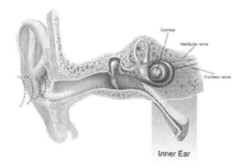

Sensorineural hearing loss is caused by a problem in the inner ear. There may be damage to the hair cells of the cochlea (which is what I have) or damage to the neural pathways of the hearing nerve. Individuals with this loss complain that they hear people talking, but do not always understand what is being said. This is because the components of sound (vowels and consonants that make up speech) are softer and distorted. I liken it to listening to a foreign language. You can hear the words but you are not able to understand what is being said.

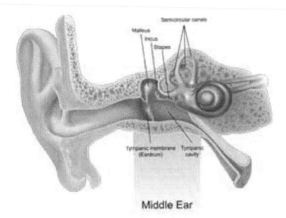

Middle Ear

Conductive Hearing Loss (CHL)

When there is a problem with sound traveling from the outer ear through the eardrum to the middle ear. That is conductive hearing loss. The manifestation of conductive hearing loss is sounds being the same, just much softer. This type of hearing loss would be closer to what you may hear if you had a cold in your head.

Causes of Hearing Loss

There are many causes of hearing loss. The Hearing Loss Association of American has a long list of potential causes.

Three common (but not all inclusive) causes for sensorineural hearing loss are:

Exposure to loud noise

Virus or disease (like my high fever that accompanied a disease)

Aging (presbycusis)

Three common (but not all inclusive) causes for conductive hearing loss are

Abnormal formation of the structure of the outer ear, ear canal, or middle ear

Fluid in the middle ear from colds or allergies or earwax

Perforated eardrum

Tinnitus

I want to address briefly Tinnitus. I do not have it, but I know SO many who do. In fact, 50 million Americans experience some degree of Tinnitus. I was stunned and amazed when delivering a talk to a group of about 30 individuals and a good quarter of them raised their hand when I asked if any of them had Tinnitus.

Tinnitus is a ringing noise in the ears when there is no actual audible noise. The intensity of the noise, I've been told by those who have it, can fluctuate. For some the Tinnitus is constant, for others it is periodic. My audiologist, who suffers from Tinnitus, offered this additional information:

"Tinnitus may be aggravated by caffeine, nicotine, excess use of alcohol, aspirin, quinine and many other medications, and stress. Different problems evaluated with Tinnitus are temporo-mandibular joint syndrome (TMJ), neck problems, allergies, and hearing loss, of course. If there is any hearing loss, the ATA (American Tinnitus Association) recommends hearing aids as they may help with Tinnitus. There are masking devices resembling hearing aids that provide sounds that help to distract from Tinnitus. I use a noisemaker in my bedroom; it is an air filter from Home Depot that makes a noise that helps to distract me from the Tinnitus."

The American Tinnitus Association offers a Tinnitus sound mixer (pictured below). A Tinnitus sufferer can pick from a variety of sounds and create a sound file that contains up to four sound elements then play the personal sound creation to mask the Tinnitus. Sort of like painting with sound. I created a sound mix of the ocean with gulls. I just love it.

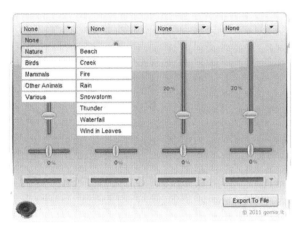

Degrees of Hearing Loss

Hearing loss is measured by the degree (severity) of the loss within frequency ranges.

Knowing the severity, type of hearing loss, and frequency range will be helpful to an audiologist and anyone else who works with people who have a hearing loss.

This next illustration shows both hearing loss range in decibels (dB) and which speech sounds and environmental sounds have become compromised.

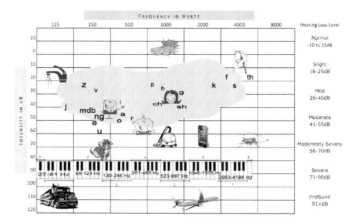

Note: The piano keyboard shows the decibel range for each octave. I cannot hear the last octave of a piano — with or without hearing aids.

Characteristics of Hearing Loss

Here are common characteristics of each of the above-mentioned degrees of loss:

Mild Hearing Loss

Mild hearing loss is a loss of approximately 25-40 decibels. People with a mild hearing loss can hear stronger vowel sounds (a, e, i, o, u) but may miss some consonant sounds that are softer (f, s, ch, th). It can sound like everyone mumbles. Consequently, they may ask people to speak louder or repeat themselves. They may find it difficult to understand soft-spoken people and young children — especially if in a noisy environment like a restaurant. People with mild hearing loss may feel like their ears are plugged or that they have wax in their ears.

Moderate Hearing Loss

Moderate hearing loss is a loss of approximately 41-55 decibels. People with moderate hearing loss have trouble hearing both consonant and vowel sounds. For example, the word "schlepp" is very difficult for me to hear and even to say. Speech comprehension becomes a challenge without hearing aids — especially if a conversation is taking place farther than 3-5 feet away. A huge percentage of a conversation may be missed if the voices are faint or if not in full view of the other person.

(Speaking from another room to a person with a moderate hearing loss is pointless).

This is the range of loss that causes people to turn up the volume on the radio or TV; so loud, it bothers others.

Moderately Severe Hearing Loss

Moderately severe hearing loss is a loss of approximately 56-70 decibels. People with moderately severe hearing loss cannot understand normal speech without some type of amplification. Without hearing aids, speech sounds like chunks of sound. When my husband sneezes from another room (a chunk of sound) I often ask, "what was that honey?" Even with hearing aids, speech may still be difficult to understand. Increasing the volume doesn't always make it clearer. Meetings and group discussions are especially challenging.

Severe Hearing Loss

Severe hearing loss is a loss of approximately 70-90 decibels. People with severe hearing loss cannot hear voices unless delivered close to the ear (from about one foot away). They cannot hear normal conversation unless it is amplified, but they can hear very loud sounds like a crying baby or barking dog.

Profound Hearing Loss

Profound hearing loss is a loss of more than 90 decibels. People with profound hearing loss may have difficulty comprehending speech even with good hearing aids. They may hear loud sounds, but more as vibrations than the actual tones. I have experienced this when an audiologist emits a tone from the audiometer that I do not HEAR, but I can FEEL. The means of communication with this degree of loss is contingent on several factors. Sign language may be an option – but with many people getting cochlear implants, it is more likely they will get hearing aids and lip read. It depends on when the hearing loss occurred. A 20-year old who develops a profound loss will likely wear hearing aids and lip read more easily than a child born with a profound hearing loss will. Additionally, how the parents have chosen to pursue education affects the means of communication; special education or regular classroom education.

My Hearing Loss

I have a combined conductive and sensorineural loss – moderate to moderately severe in the right ear and moderately severe to severe in my left. My loss was due, primarily, to that high fever when I was four years old. However, for millions of Americans, adult-onset hearing loss is due to noise. More on that in another chapter.[1]

Treating Hearing Loss

For individuals who have severe to profound hearing loss, cochlear, or brain stem implants are a possibility. However, by NO means do these treatments restore one to perfect hearing. I listened to an example of what sound is like via a cochlear implant. It is like listening to a conversation or music from the bottom of a six-foot deep pool. I never LOVED what hearing I have until I heard that sample. The sound samples are on YouTube.

The most common treatment for hearing loss is hearing aids. Again, they do not restore one to the hearing they enjoyed prior to the loss. Nevertheless, they will help one stay connected. We will examine hearing aids more closely in an upcoming chapter[2]

In conclusion:

There are two basic types of hearing loss — sensorineural and conductive. Sensorineural loss affects the inner ear while conductive loss affects the middle or outer ear. There are several causes for the loss, and varying degrees of loss. The ability to comprehend speech depends on the type and severity of the loss. The important distinction between sensorineural hearing loss and conductive hearing loss is that conductive may be medically treated. Profound sensorineural hearing loss can be treated with cochlear implants. By and large, most hearing loss is treated with hearing aids.

Chapter 4 References and Resources.

---

[1]See Chapter: How to Damage Your Hearing
[2] See Chapter: Hearing Aids – the Saving Grace – the Necessary Evil

Hearing Loss Association. (n.d).. *Types, causes and treatment*. Retrieved January 2014, from Hearing Loss Association of America: .http://www.hearingloss.org/content/types-causes-and-treatment

American Tinnitus Association. (n.d).. *Sound* . Retrieved October 2014, from American Tinnitus Association: http://www.ata.org/sound

You tube video created by sensimetrics.com that provides sample of what speech and music sounds like with cochlear implants:

http://www.youtube.com/watch?v=SpKKYBkJ9Hw.

CHAPTER 5:
HOW TO DAMAGE YOUR HEARING

"I have unwittingly helped to invent and refine a type of music that makes its principal components deaf. Hearing loss is a terrible thing because it cannot be repaired." – Pete Townshend

In the previous chapter, we learned of two primary types of hearing loss and their causes: conductive and sensorineural. At the top of the list for the cause of sensorineural loss are loud noises. It is the most common cause of Tinnitus. Loud music is what caused rock star Pete Townshend to lose his hearing. Not just on stage, but via headphones during studio sessions.

How Loud is Too Loud?

The loudness or intensity of sound is measured in decibels (dBs). The capital B is for the founder of this measurement, Alexander Graham Bell. I compiled the chart below from a variety of resources on the Internet. The chart shows common sounds and their average dB level. When sound reaches about 100 decibels, it can be painful and we have to cover our ears.

DB Range	SOUND	DB Range	SOUND
20-30	Ticking watch, bedroom at night	110-120	Blow dryer, subway train, MP3 players, sirens, ambulance
30-40	Quiet whisper, library, rice Krispies in milk	120-130	Power mower, chainsaw, firecracker, fire alarm
40-50	Refrigerator hum, speech	130-140	Screaming Child
50-60	Rainfall, quiet restaurant dining	120	Thunderclap
60-70	Sewing Machine, shower,	120-139	Sport events, Rock concert
70-80	Washing Machine, electric shaver, TV average	130-140	Jackhammer, jet plane, gunshot
80-90	Alarm Clock (2 ft. away) lawn mower, piano, symphony concert	160	Grenade
90-100	Average traffic, electric drill, electric dryer, garbage disposal, Bulldozer, night clubs, many noise making children toys	170	Airbag
100-110	MP3 players, snowmobile, motorcycles, helicopter take off	180-190	Rocket Launch, Call of the Blue Whale

When Is Our Hearing At Risk?

85 dB, according to United States Department of Labor – Occupational Safety and Health Administration, is a level that causes hearing damage. Not all loud sounds will result in hearing loss; it depends on the intensity and duration of the noise. Prolonged exposure to sounds exceeding 80 decibels (dB) can result in permanent hearing loss.

Given this, it is a good practice to wear earplugs when exposed to sound 85 dB and above – that means, when you are vacuuming or using a leaf blower! The table below reflects which decibel levels can cause hearing damage over a period of time. Some damage is immediate. Damage can be temporary or permanent. These numbers are based on the findings from the National Institute of Occupational Safety and Health (NIOSH).

85 dB	8 hours	100 dB	15 minutes
88 dB	4 hours	115 dB	15 seconds
91 dB	2 hours	120 dB	8 seconds
94 dB	60 minutes	140+ dB	immediate
97 dB	30 minutes		

I have created a PDF of this little table that you can print or share with others and it you can obtain it on my Hearing Loss Tips website.

I recently learned that a man was standing next to an angry percussionist who slammed a large gong with the hammer. The sound pierced his ears in pain and when the pain subsided, there was a ringing, which, four years later, continues. He is finding it increasingly difficult hear women in social situations. A tragic occurrence.

There are several Smartphone decibel meter apps so you can easily check the decibel level of your environment, a piece of machinery, a toy, an MP3 player, etc. Below is an example of one I have on my Android phone called the Sound Meter. It is free and available in Google Play.

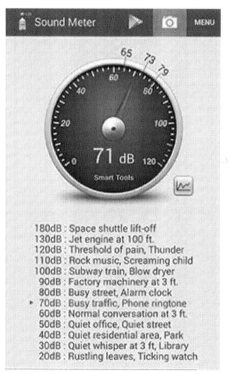

This reading was taken at a restaurant where I was having breakfast.

I like the simple guidance provided by the American Tinnitus Association.

If you cannot understand what someone is saying 3 feet away from you, the noise level could be harming your hearing.

I have also heard that if you need to raise your voice in a noisy environment, the noise could be harming your hearing.

Hearing loss in children

I recently attended a GLAD (Greater Los Angeles Agency on Deafness) open house. I met a hearing specialist who shared that she is seeing more incidences of children with noise induced hearing loss.

The toy manufacturers are partly to blame. Many toys make noise at a level of 100 decibels or more. The American Society for Testing and Materials International, ASTM, has established that a safe limit for children's toys is 85 decibels at 40 centimeters (about 20 inches) away from the child's ears. Next time you go shopping for toys take along your Smartphone with a decibel meter on it and test the volume level of toys before purchasing them.

Protecting a baby's hearing

What do you do when taking a baby somewhere that you know is dangerously loud? A woman I know owns a roller skate shop and frequently has a booth at roller-derby events. These events are ROWDY NOISY. Having struggled with tinnitus in one of her ears for most of her adult life, she does not wish the same curse on her newborn baby boy. She invested in hearing protection earmuffs for infants. Her baby boy fussed a bit with them on, but certainly not enough to have to remove them. Here he is wearing them:

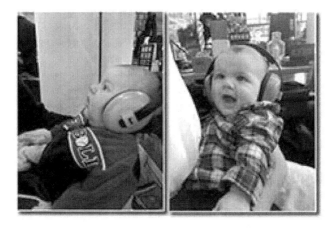

Two manufacturers of hearing protection earmuffs for infants and children are Banz and EM's for Children.

Live sound is not the only cause of hearing loss

Interestingly enough, Pete Townshend says the cause of his type of hearing loss was not so much playing loud music on stage as it was using headphones in the recording studio.

The average listening level of MP3 players is 100 – 110 decibels. Over time, that is going to damage hearing.

There are many makers of noise-reduction headphones for kids that restrict the volume level, no matter how loud the volume is turned up. Search "noise reduction headphones" in Google and take your pick.

For teens and adults, it is up to the listener to protect his or her hearing by not blasting sound through headsets directly into the ears. On my Smartphone, I get this warning when I try to turn up the volume of my headset:

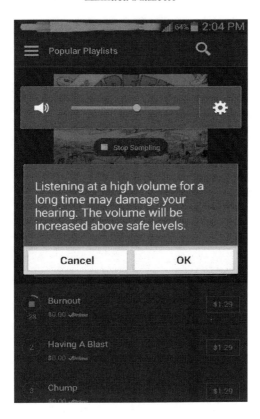

During my youth, I did stupid things that likely further damaged my hearing. Most memorable was a rock concert whereby my body felt transparent as the sound boomed through. My ears felt "spongy" for FOUR days following that concert.

I also used to listen to music through headphones so loud my parents could hear it across the room.

No one could convince me to protect what hearing I had. No one.

Perhaps having some knowledge of what it is like to have a hearing loss may inspire you or someone you love to protect her or his ears. There are plenty of sobering sound samples on the web.[3]

In conclusion:

Noise can damage your hearing regardless of the source. Protect your

---

[3] See Chapter: What is it Like to Live With a Hearing Loss

ears. The easiest way to do that is to listen to music at a lower volume through headphones and to wear earplugs or earmuffs when exposed to sound levels exceeding 90-100 decibels.

However, if you are already experiencing diminished hearing, not all is lost, yet. As you will see in the next chapter, you can get your ears tested to find out how minor or major your loss is and what to do about it.

Chapter 5 References and Resources:

NIOSH. (June, 1998). *Criteria For a Recommended Standard - Occupational Noise Exposure.* Washington, DC: US Department of Health and Human Services.

NIOSH. (n.d).. *Office of Mine Safety and Health Research (OMSHR).* Retrieved from Centers for Disease Control and Prevention: http://www.cdc.gov/niosh/mining/works/coversheet1820.html

Standard Consumer Safety Specification forToy Safety. (n.d).. Retrieved October 17, 2014, from American Society for Testing and Materials (ASTM): http://www.astm.org/DATABASE.CART/HISTORICAL/F963-08.htm

Amazon. (2006, January 5). *US Showbiz.* Retrieved June 16, 2014, from Mail Online: http://www.dailymail.co.uk/tvshowbiz/article-373283/Townshend-warning-iPod-users.html

Linnaea Mallette

CHAPTER 6:
DO YOU HAVE A HEARING LOSS?

"When someone in the family has a hearing loss, the whole family has a hearing problem."
– Dr. Mark Ross

A delightful woman in one of my Toastmaster clubs gave a speech about when she realized she had a hearing problem; while serving on Jury duty…

"It was then I first realized I was going deaf. I **could** hear the Lawyer and I **could** hear the witness/ But I couldn't hear the judge! It was a drunken driving case and fortunately, I was an alternate. Everything was going fine until the judge turned to us and said: 'Now I want you to…&#%!@?!…; and then &#%!@?! *….' I looked at the other jurors and they were nodding, like they knew what she was saying. Fortunately, the case was adjudicated. Thankfully, I was not called on to make a decision."

A subsequent visit to an audiologist revealed she had a moderate hearing loss.

The National Institute on Deafness and Other Communication Disorders (NIDCD) offers this simple test to determine if you may have a hearing loss. If you answer "yes" to three or more of the questions, it is time to have your hearing checked

Here are some of the most common indicators I have noticed:

Everyone seems to mumble

Constantly asking people to repeat themselves

Being told the TV (or radio) is too loud

Every phone call seems like a bad connection.

"Everyone mumbles!"

"What?"   "Pardon me?"

"Turn down the TV!"

"We must have a bad   "Huh?"
connection..."

Getting Your Ears Tested

Audiologist or Hearing Instrument Specialist?

When getting your ears tested make sure, you get as comprehensive an evaluation as possible, and an objective presentation of the aids best suited for your loss and your budget. If possible, visit an audiologist, not a hearing specialist or hearing aid dealers. The primary reason is education.

Generally, hearing instrument specialists must have at least a high school diploma or GED with a certain number of hours in supervised training where they practice giving hearing tests, making ear molds, and fitting hearing aids. They are limited to testing and fitting of aids only. They do not diagnose the cause of the hearing loss.

On the other hand, to be an audiologist, one must have a Doctoral degree from an accredited university graduate program in audiology; acceptance into an audiology program is very stringent. Audiologists are qualified and trained to assess the reasons/causes behind hearing loss and treat or rehabilitate the loss. If necessary, they refer cases for appropriate medical or surgical treatment (such as treatment for a conductive hearing loss or cochlear implants).

Here are the qualifications of my audiologist who works at Audiology

Associates in Santa Clarita, California:

"Patrice received her Master's Degree in Audiology from California State University, Northridge in 1995 and her Doctorate from the University of Florida in 2004. She is licensed by the state in Audiology and hearing aid dispensing. Patrice holds certifications of clinical competence from the American Speech and Hearing Association and the American Academy of Audiology. She also holds teaching credentials in special education and taught in the Santa Clarita Valley elementary schools for 10 years. She has lived in the SCV with her family for over 20 years. Her professional affiliations include the American Speech and Hearing Association, American Academy of Audiology, California Academy of Audiology, and American Hearing Aid Associates."

This woman knows her stuff. More importantly, she is a CARING audiologist. I don't care HOW educated a person is, if he/she isn't caring and sensitive, I'm not interested!

Now don't get me wrong. I'm not implying that a hearing instrument specialist should be avoided at all cost. What I am saying is that an audiologist has been trained to diagnose your hearing loss and make sure you get the type of aids programmed that will best suit your type of hearing loss. I know of many hearing instrument specialists that have delivered exemplary service to those who visited them. As with any service provider, some are better than others are. That goes for hearing instrument specialists and audiologists alike.

Let me share with you my recommendations based on my own personal experience when it comes to finding the right professional/organization to take care of my hearing problems.

Things to Consider

Check your insurance. It may have coverage for hearing loss testing and hearing aids. BUT, a word of caution here, I had that with my medical coverage. However, the hearing tests and dispensing of aids were available only with a specific dealer. Years later I found out, by accident, that this dealer had a special relationship with one of the major hearing aid manufacturers in the country, so I was never offered any other type of hearing aids. AND I was never told about those extra perks available with Bluetooth, streamers, etc.

The ONLY way I found out about my current aids (by Oticon) and the available accessories was by conversing with a woman who recently was fitted with aids and technology similar to what I now have. I went back to the dealer I was limited to due to my type of insurance coverage and asked why they never told me about these other type of aids and technology. The audiologist was pretty "cool" in her response. I left in a huff and never went back. The real kicker is this: The insurance coverage offered $1,100 per aid, every 3 years. Yet, the private audiologist I now have was able to meet that reduced price WITHOUT INSURANCE.

Ask for a referral: Once I found out about the type of aids and devices available, a friend gave me a referral. I visited the audiologist and was surprised at the difference in service. Friends or family may know of audiologists that they or people they know with whom they have been pleased.

Distance: Fortunately, the referral did not require me to drive more than 30 minutes in traffic to reach the audiologist. Ideally, you want to find an audiologist that does not require hours of driving to get back and forth. You will be visiting the audiologist for annual hearing tests, and more often, to have ear molds cleaned and tubing replaced.

History: Consider a business with a history of at least 20-30 years. This was not one of my criteria, but one must agree that usually a company or individual who has been in business successfully for 20-30 years is doing something right. (I have since found out that my audiologist has been in business 19 years as of 2014).

Caring, unrushed attention: This is *so important*. I NEVER felt special at the dealer attached to my insurance coverage. In addition to not getting objective recommendations, I felt like an object moving down the assembly line. This is NOT how I feel with my current audiologist. She is sensitive. Patient. I never feel rushed. And I feel special. That means a lot to me. Hearing loss is problematic enough without dealing with a cold machine-like audiologist or worst, used-car-salesman type of hearing instrument specialist at a hearing aid dealer.

The Hearing Examination

Once you have found your audiologist or specialist, you need to get your hearing tested. Let's examine a little more closely, what you may expect during the hearing examination (based on my personal experience and under the care of an audiologist).

When I go for testing, there are usually four or five hearing tests performed:

1. The Audiometer test
2. Bone Conduction Hearing test
3. Hearing with Noise test
4. Speech Recognition test
5. Speech Discrimination test

During my last visit, my audiologist performed two additional tests I had never undertaken before:

6. Tympanometry test
7. Acoustic reflexes test

All the tests — except the tympanometry and acoustic reflexes test — were performed in a small quiet soundproof room (photograph below). The other two were performed in an open room.

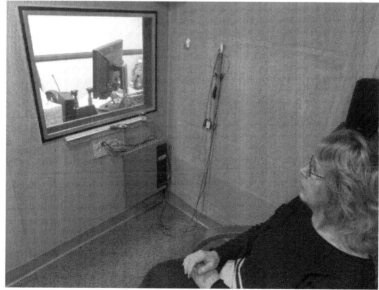

Audiometer Test

An audiometer is used to determine hearing sensitivity at different frequencies. It includes not only volume (soft to loud) but also frequencies (low to high). The audiologist either places headphones over the ears or inserts earphones into the ear canals. In my case, earphones were used. I push a button or raise my hand when I hear a sound made by the audiometer. Sounds are delivered at different frequencies. As I respond, my audiologist marks the results on an audiogram.

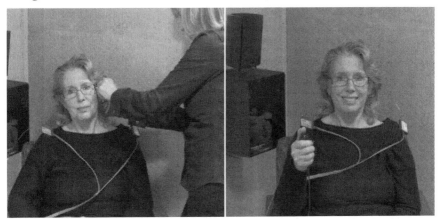

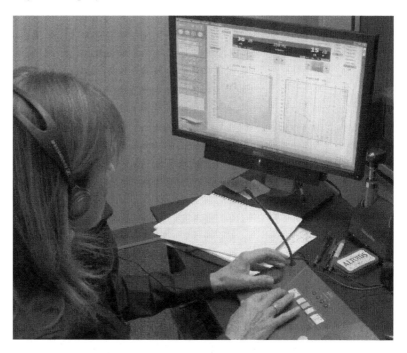

The sounds that occur above the jagged plotted lines are the ones I have difficulty hearing and sounds below the lines are what I can hear. Here is my audiogram from a hearing test conducted January 2014:

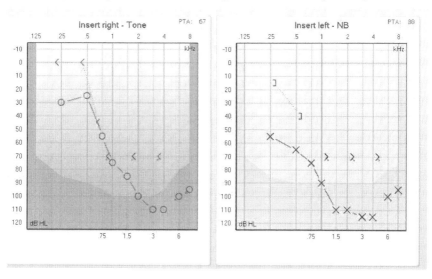

Sometimes the right and left ear are plotted on the same graph. In my case, the left and right ears have graphs of their own. The circle represents the right ear; the X represents the left ear. The bone conduction test results are represented by ">" for the left year and "<" for the right ear. A visual representation of this loss in different environments and for speech appears in a later chapter.[4]

Bone Conduction Hearing Test

The Bone Conduction hearing test helps my audiologist determine the type of hearing loss I may have. Is it sensorineural? Conductive? A combination of both? For this test, my audiologist placed a small vibrator on the bone behind my ear (the vibrator could be placed on the forehead). Once again, I push a button or raise my hand when I hear something.

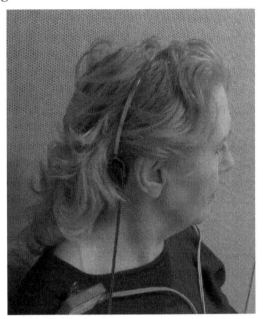

Hearing in Noise Test

In this test, the audiologist tests how well I hear sounds and understand speech while there is background noise. The background

---

[4] See Chapter: What is it Like to Have a Hearing Loss?

noise is called "white noise" or "speech noise."

Speech-Recognition and Understanding Tests

The speech recognition test involves words, not tones, from an audiometer. It is conducted in that little soundproof room also. During this test, the audiologist asks me to repeat the words she says. I usually feel silly during this test because so many words are just chunks of sound; often I take a feeble stab at what the word might be. Here is a very simplistic example the audiologist says to me:

"Say the word 'bye'" – I respond.
"Say the word 'lye'" – I respond.
"Say the word 'nice'" – I respond.
"Say the word 'hike'" – I respond.
...and so forth.

By performing this test, my audiologist can better understand my communication challenges since the test reveals what components of speech I do or do not comprehend.

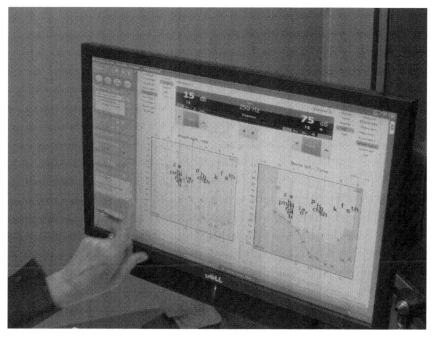

See the results of my speech recognition test. The sounds below the line, I hear. Sounds above the line, I do not hear. As you can see, my hearing loss is a bit complex when it comes to speech.

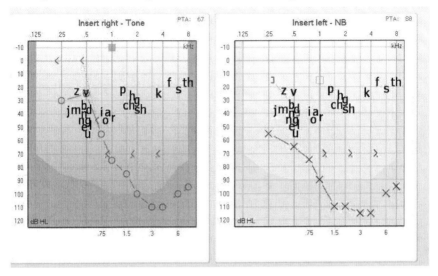

Once finished with the tests in the soundproof room, I am escorted to another area with a big chair that sort of resembles a dentist's chair. There, two more tests are conducted.

Tympanometry Test

A tympanometry test checks the condition of the middle ear. That is, how well my eardrums move and how well the bones are conducting. A device that looked like a probe is held to my ears, one at a time, and the function of the eardrum is detected by its response to the air pressure caused by the probe. The test lasts just seconds and is not uncomfortable.

Acoustic Reflexes Test

The acoustic reflexes test checks the bones in the middle ear by emitting a loud sound at a few frequencies and gauging the response of the middle ear. If there is no reflex, it may indicate a problem with the bones. The tests revealed my bones were not moving as much as they could, but the problem was not super severe.

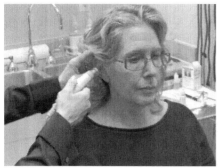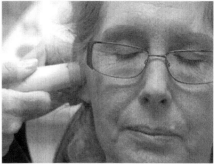

The conclusion after all the tests were completed is that I have a combination of sensorineural and conductive hearing loss with a moderate to moderately severe loss in the right here and a moderately severe to severe loss in the left ear.

A full hearing examination like this can take anywhere from 45-90 minutes. The results help an audiologist select and program the hearing aids.loss.

In conclusion:

If you believe you have a hearing loss, seek a qualified, caring audiologist or hearing specialist to conduct your hearing tests and recommend hearing aids most suitable for your loss (and budget).

Chapter 6 References and Resources:

Video of talk given by Barbara Massey about her hearing loss and challenges with the TV

http://www.youtube.com/watch?v=QXEmsEs8bHM&feature=youtu.be

NIDCD. (n.d).. *Ten Ways To Recognize Hearing Loss.* Retrieved from National Institute on Deafness and Other Communication Disorders: http://www.nidcd.nih.gov/health/hearing/pages/10ways.aspx

Audiology Associates: http://www.audiologyassociates.net

Linnaea Mallette

CHAPTER 7:
HEARING AIDS – THE SAVING GRACE – THE NECESSARY EVIL

I CAN HEAR!!! It is completely life changing and emotional! For those of you who thought I was ignoring you or just blonde... I promise you our relationship will go to new levels. It's kind of cute but you cannot see it, just a teeny clear plastic wire. But I kinda feel like Mel Gibson in What Women Want...I hear EVERYTHING! This being able to hear stuff takes some getting used to.... —Sally Van Swearingen, Owner of The A-List hair and makeup studio, Santa Clarita, CA

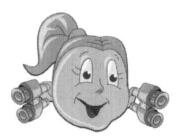

I love this quote from Dr. Cynthia Compton Connelly: *"Assistive listening devices are like binoculars for the ears."*

I believe she is talking about the BENEFIT of hearing aids. That is, amplifying – making bigger – sounds we do not hear. From my perspective as an aid wearer, I interpret the quote to mean hearing aids being as obtrusive and visible as having binoculars sticking out of my ears. Obviously, hearing aids are not binoculars, so exactly what are they?

What is a Hearing Aid?

A hearing aid is a device worn in the ear to amplify sounds. It is sort of like an audio set up at a conference. There are three basic components:

a microphone, amplifier, and speaker. When a person speaks into the microphone, it converts the sound into electrical signals and sends them to an amplifier. The amplifier increases the power of the signals and sends them through the speaker out into the audience. Compress those three components into a small compartment, add a battery, and you have a hearing aid. Only, the hearing aid is not amplifying the sound out into an audience. It is amplifying the sound right into your ear.

There are many hearing aid types and styles.

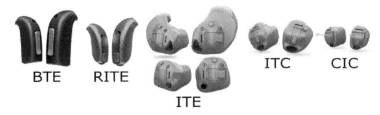

BTE   RITE   ITE   ITC   CIC

BTE – A Behind the Ear hearing aid is housed in a small curved case that fits behind the ear. It is attached to an ear mold created from an impression of your outer ear. The case is usually an unobtrusive flesh color but can be purchased in many colors and/or patterns. This is the type of aid I wear.

RITE – The receiver in the ear model is a newer development in hearing aids and is suitable for mild to severe hearing loss. The receiver or speaker is placed in the ear with a soft tip. There is still a casing behind the ear, but it is smaller than the BTE style. This is the most common type of hearing aid fit now.

ITE – An In the Ear hearing aid fits directly into the external ear.

ITC – An In the Canal hearing aid is so small it can fill just a small portion of the external ear.

CIC – A Completely in the Canal hearing aid is nearly invisible as it fits deeply into the ear canal.

Most hearing aids today are only available in digital format. I believe one can purchase used or refurbished analog aids. Digital is the standard, and for very good reasons!

Analog aids amplify a sound wave by simply making it larger. The choices in programming are "louder" or "softer." That's it.

Digital aids, however, take the incoming signal from the microphone and convert it into a digital format. The beauty of digital aids is that they are programmable. There is much more flexibility in adjusting the way the aid "hears" to the benefit and comfort of the wearer. Picture an equalizer where you can adjust several different frequencies, at different levels – soft, medium and loud input. The audiologist can adjust MANY levels of sound this way to help you hear better and more comfortably!

Take me for example. I have two Oticon "Chili" BTEs. After all the hearing tests were done, my audiologist hooked up my aids to the computer by hanging a wireless hearing aid connector called a "near-com" around my neck. She asked a series of lifestyle questions to create a personalized program for me.

Here is how they were programmed:

Hearing in a normal environment – home, work, driving, etc.

Restaurant setting – mutes background noise and focuses on the person in front of me.

Music setting – all channels open so I can enjoy full range of music that I am able to perceive.

Phone setting – the "telecoil" that amplifies speech on the phone[5]

On the follow-up visit she reviewed the data the hearing aids had collected over the last six months. She could tell I wore the aids on an average of seven hours a day. She could tell I often turn them down low. When asked why, I told her, "Things are just too loud."

---

[5] See Chapter: Additional Assistive Devices and Technology

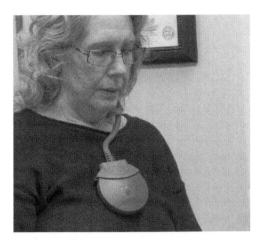

My Audiologist could see I did not use the fourth setting so she offered to remove it. Then, while discussing the squeaking of the aides and the volume information she saw in the software, she asked a few pertinent questions to understand better the type of hearing environments I most often find myself.

I told her that as an active leader within Toastmasters and a professional speaker, I am often in conference settings – and can't hear well! My audiologist changed that fourth setting to a "conference" setting. It is more severe than the restaurant setting in that it blocks out much more of the background noise and amplifies, even more, the person in front of me.

She also adjusted the "noise" level of the first setting, just a tad. Without compromise to the range of amplification needed for speech comprehension, the optimal volume was changed for a more comfortable, and less "squeaky setting."

The Saving Grace

The flexibility in programming with digital aids, and the psychological and relationship benefits discussed in an upcoming chapter[6] do make hearing aids a saving grace. They are a far better choice than withdrawal and depression!

I am often tempted to say the "evils" of hearing aids outweigh the

---

[6] See Chapter: What is it Like to Live with a Hearing Loss?

benefit…but truth be told, I'd be LOST without my precious hearing aids. In the best of environments, my speech comprehension in my right ear is 60% and only 27% in my left ear. When I do not wear my hearing aids, my speech comprehension is immediately impacted and people around me have to repeat themselves several times before I can understand what they are saying. Close friends have told me that they can tell I am not wearing my aids because my *own* speech is not as clear. Without my aids, I have to work 10 times harder to hear. Without my aids, I can enjoy quiet, but not connection.

I am a visitor and occasional contributor to a wonderful website called "Hearing Like Me" which is a community for those who have been touched by hearing loss. One of the Ambassadors of the site that goes by the name "Streamer" shared a great deal about his own experience with hearing loss. With his permission, I am sharing what he had to say about his discovery of the benefit of hearing aids. This man was not diagnosed with a loss until in the fourth grade. In addition, at that time, he was told there weren't any aids that could treat his level of loss, but hearing aids would be in his future. Here is his story:

"…That future turned out to be a little over 40 years later. One day I asked my sister to try on her hearing aids, could not believe what I was missing, and went in for a much-needed hearing test about a week later. At the time the audiologist told me I must have lost my hearing after I had learned to talk or I would talk like a deaf person and I must have the ability to determine what people are saying even though I only hear pieces of the words because my word recognition scores were very — and are very — good.

After getting hearing aids I soon realized I probably should have gotten them about 10 years earlier because my life became much easier with them than without them. People always said I talked too loud and at the end of the day my tongue would actually be sore from talking too loud. Once I got hearing aids, people would comment that I didn't speak as loudly as I once did and wanted to know what happened and once I told them that I was now wearing hearing aids, they couldn't believe it could make that much of a difference. Another benefit was not having to ask people to repeat what they had said as often and I'm sure it made other people's lives easier as well.

Another unforeseen benefit to wearing hearing aids has been a significant reduction in my tinnitus. Most of the time during the day, for all intent and purposes, it is basically gone while I am wearing my hearing aids and at the end of the day when I remove my HA's it is diminished in its intensity and gradually comes back during the night as I sleep."

For me, having and wearing hearing aids is a no brainer.

However, that does not preclude me from sharing the necessary evil aspects of hearing aids, to be grounded in the reality of wearing aids. Studies show that only one in five people who need hearing aids wear them. One of the reasons is denial they even need them. The other is what I call the "Necessarily Evil" factors of hearing aids.

The Necessary Evil

I wear two BTE aids attached to a custom earpiece. While I appreciate the HELP my hearing aids provide, they really are a pain in the neck. I find myself frequently complaining about them aloud or to myself. Here are some of the things I dislike about hearing aids. These are not in order of discontent. Their order of importance depends on my mood and the circumstances under which they are not behaving.

They Are Not Pretty

I have hair that covers my ears, so it really doesn't matter what color the aids are. Though mine are flesh colored, aids do come in choices of colors depending on the manufacturer. One of them, Naida, has 18 colors – including a zebra and giraffe pattern!

I do know that some aids are designed to resemble a wireless Bluetooth headset, which can prevent the challenge of an aid that is visible to the public. I think this is a good choice for a junior high or high school student to ward off teasing.

There are crafts people creating jewelry specifically designed to be worn on hearing aids (they clip onto or hang from the hearing aid tubing). These can make wearing hearing aids more attractive, even flashy and fashionable. Circe Denyer made me a pair of hearing aid charms with cats because I love cats. She sells these on Etsy.

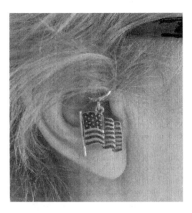

Visibility

When the aids are visible, some people treat me weirdly or avoid me altogether. This can be a benefit in some cases (as described in the Benefits chapter[7]). At the other extreme, people assume I can hear normally and do not make an effort to make sure I am hearing them (more on this later under "myths")[8].

Amplification

Aids amplify everything. Digital aids can help minimize the cacophony of amplified sounds, but they do not completely solve the challenge.

Discomfort

Aids make my ears ache after wearing them for 12 hours or more. In fact, my ears are so sensitive that if I wear them 12 hours or more a day for 2-3 days in a row, I usually get a mild outer ear infection. When I travel to conferences or trips, I take a small bottle of prescribed eardrops just in case. My audiologist suggested I try lubricating the ear molds with baby oil or mineral oil. I'll try that.

Feedback

A squealing/whistling sound is a frequent embarrassment for me. It only happens when the aids are confined, that is, do not have much

---

[7] See Chapter: Benefits of Hearing Loss
[8] See Chapter: Hearing Loss Myths

breathing space. For me it happens in elevators and when I hug someone. In elevators, people are alarmed wondering if there is something happening to the elevator. I apologize and explain, pointing at my ears, that my piglets are squealing. It puts people at ease and lessens my embarrassment. This squealing is not normal for most wearers. It is for me because of the way the molds completely and snugly fit in my ear and the power of my aids; both given the severity of my loss.

Batteries

Aids run on batteries, which seem to go dead at the most inconvenient times. My aids beep when the batteries are beginning to go dead, so I can excuse myself to a private place and change the batteries. I draw much unwanted attention to myself if I change the aids in the presence of others. What I do now is change the batteries if it has been a while and I am about to enter into a long day or evening social event.

Maintenance

The ear molds can get sticky if one's ear produces a lot of wax, like mine. I should wipe them down each night when I take them off, but I don't. The tubing should be changed every three months as it hardens and affects the flow of sound from the ear mold to the ear. My provider does this as a complimentary service (as well as providing hearing aid batteries).

Cost

AIDS ARE EXPENSIVE! The most recent pair I purchased cost me over $6,000 - $3,000 each. Cost is probably the #1 reason why people don't invest in hearing aids. Consumer Reports cited the hearing aids they tested ranged from $1,800 to $7,200 per pair. I financed my aids via a credit service, which allowed me 12 months to pay the balance in full with no finance charge. Wherever you purchase your aids, I'm sure there is a payment plan of some sort available to you.

Because hearing aids are SO expensive, I always purchase hearing aid insurance too. Usually aids are covered automatically the first year after purchase; thereafter, the insurance runs anywhere from $100 - $200 a year. It is best to ask the hearing aid provider for the actual cost. Part of the cost of hearing aids includes the complimentary supply of batteries, hearing aid cleaning and tubes changed. When I return to the office for adjustments or cleaning, there is no additional cost.

I go in every 3 months to have my tubing changed and pick up additional packs of hearing aid batteries. So that's 4 visits a year times probably 6 years before I get new hearing aids. If I had to pay for the batteries and tube changes on my own, that would add up to a considerable amount of money. Before I learned I had insurance to cover for the cost of hearing aids, I paid $50.00 to have my tubes changed per visit. Because it was so expensive I didn't do it very often, which meant I didn't hear as well as I could have. Tubes that are hardened do not transmit sound well to the receiver.

Warning to New Users

Hearing aids assist, but they do NOT restore the perfect hearing you once enjoyed.

Most of the people I know who wear hearing aids do not have "normal" hearing when wearing them. I sure don't. In fact, at times they interfere with what hearing I do have.

Individuals who need hearing aids have to realize that the aids will help, but the expectation that they will once again enjoy the hearing they once had will lead to a devastating disappointment. I personally know a nice guy who experienced this. I'll call him Alex for the purpose of this chapter.

Alex had Tinnitus for years and years. It seriously affected his hearing. The common response individuals who suffer from this get from specialists and audiologists is, "hearing aids can't help you." Therefore, Alex had gone for most of his adult life (he is in his 60's) before he accompanied his girlfriend to hear me speak at a local chapter of a hearing loss association. There he met an audiologist who told him she believed she COULD help him. And she did. She was able to fit him with aids.

So Alex eagerly awaited the arrival of the aids fully expecting, really believing, they were going to restore his hearing to what he enjoyed as a young adult.

When I saw Alex several months later, I inquired as to how he was doing with his aids. His eyes misted up. His voice had the tone of hurtful disappointment and frustration, *"...I expected to have perfect hearing again...."* I so identified with his response. The painful truth is, as Alex discovered, hearing aids help, but they do not restore one to normal hearing.

Hearing Aid Guidance for the New User

While researching for the weekly blog posts on my hearing loss site, I found a most wonderful resource for individuals new to the hearing aid experience. The resource is an article by researcher Dr. Mark Ross who is himself hard of hearing.

I had some of these experiences when I first got hearing aids. Many of them echo what Dr. Ross shares in his article.

SOUNDS

It took time for me to adjust to the way my environment sounded through the hearing aids. Dr. Ross likens it to getting used to understanding someone who has an accent. It takes time for the brain to re-educate itself in interpreting the sounds as they come through the hearing aid.

I heard sounds I had not ever heard before. It was alarming to hear all sounds that I did not recognize. I recall being alarmed at the sound of the hum of the refrigerator. I had NEVER heard the hum of a refrigerator. Another alarming sound was the clicking of my turn indicator in my car. I thought something was wrong with the car.

ACCLIMATING TO AIDS

When I first got hearing aids and wore them everywhere, I got very agitated and eventually quite depressed. It was too much to process all at once mentally and emotionally. I was constantly adjusting the volume on my aids depending on where I was. Before long, I had no idea what my "true north" was for my hearing aid setting. I became even more depressed at the amount of work it took to wear the darn aids.

So, for me, I had to get used to the aids bit by bit. Dr. Ross says it takes about 3-4 weeks to get used to what life sounds like through hearing aids. Professionals call this the acclimatization period and the main reason hearing aids are fit for a 30-day trial. It took a while, but eventually I figured out what works for me and what doesn't and adjusting the aids accordingly eventually became second nature. It helped tremendously to make a note of which situations were most challenging for me and share them with my audiologist. She was able to make adjustments to the aids to suit my comfort level. Conversely, as I got more and more used to the hearing aids and my comfort level changed, the settings on the hearing aids were often subsequently adjusted.

THE TINNY SOUND

In the beginning, I was very unhappy with the "tinny" sound of speech and had that band of sound (high frequencies) turned down and the low frequencies turned up. In time, when I got used to the aids, I had the high frequencies brought back as I realized that the "tinny" sounds are part of what makes up the components of speech. I was not able to understand conversation as well with the high frequencies turned down as I could with them turned up.

PATIENCE

The recommendation I would make to anyone first getting hearing aids is to be patient and give it time. Go slow. Make notes and keep in touch with your audiologist or hearing specialist. Please, do read Dr. Ross's outstanding discourse on this topic of wearing aids for the first time. In fact, the experiences I expressed above are pretty much, what I go through every time I get a new pair of hearing aids!

Ten ways to get the most out of your hearing aid investment

The hearing aids are a hefty financial investment. Here are some tips I have learned (often the hard way) to get the most out of that investment:

1. **Keep your hearing aids away from pets**. Pets like hearing aids! I had a cat that LOVED licking the wax off my ear molds. So if my aids were anywhere out in the open, in the morning they would be on the floor clean as a whistle. Fortunately, I did not ever step on them. But I or my husband sure could have! I have heard from others that they have had some serious hearing aid damage when their dog got ahold of one. So, keep those aids in a cabinet or drawer where a pet cannot access them.

2. **Keep aids away from toddlers and children**: They may be curious, but your aids are very fragile and they may not know what "careful" means. Keep them in your ears or out of sight of the young ones when not wearing them.

3. **Don't put hearing aids on until after you are done applying make-up and fussing with your hair.** Hair spray and make-up can clog up the microphone. If that happens, you will need to pay a visit to the audiologist to get the aid(s) fixed.

4. **Avoid melting your hearing aid.** Hearing aids are encased in plastic. Plastic melts. I once hung my hearing aids on a lampshade. Yes, the heat of the light bulb melted the aids. Having aids close to cooking appliances is not a good idea. You may wonder how one could have an aid close to an appliance? Easy! The phone rings while in the kitchen or outside Barbequing, you take off the aid, lay it down, and forget about it.

5. **Don't let the tubing get too hard.** I was NEVER told, until I acquired the services of my newest audiologist, that the tubing on aids should be changed every 2-3 months for maximum effectiveness. Why? As the tubes harden, the sound passing through bounces off the walls compromising the quality of the sound passing into the aid. Time flies, I often forget. But when I suddenly realize I just can't hear that well with the aids, I check the tubing! More often than not, they are stiff.

6. **Change the batteries often.** With my latest aids, when the batteries are dying I get a beeping noise. Prior to these aids, I did not have that feature, and the aids would slowly die, meaning the quality of hearing dissipated. I often did not notice that until the battery went completely dead. I cannot tell you how often to change your batteries as it depends on the type of

battery, how often you wear your aids, how loud, and for how long. Check with your audiologist or hearing aid specialist.

7. **Keep the aids dry.** Exposure to too much moisture can harm the electrical parts of a hearing aid. I store mine in my bathroom where I take a bath, but they are in a container that resists moisture. Take care when sweating a lot. I do not wear my aids when I am exercising. However, I do wear them in the heat of the Southern California summer and I sweat. You can purchase what is called a drying kit to wick that moisture away from the aids.

8. **Check and double-check your ears.** Get into the habit of checking your ears any time you step into a shower, bath or pool. The day will come when you are so used to wearing your aids you will forget you are wearing them. I always stick my fingers in my ears before I hop into the shower or dive into the ocean to make sure I have my aids off.

9. **Keep aids from getting too cold.** I do not have this problem. I live in Southern California. However, those who live in the extreme cold, guard the aids. I find that a sock hat goes nicely over my aids and doesn't cause feedback. Extreme cold (or hot) can cause the casing to melt or crack and the digital chip can be harmed. No digital chip, no aids.

10. **Don't lose your aids.** My audiologist indicated that the danger of taking an aid off to talk on the phone is walking off and leaving it behind. I usually try to stay conscious and put the aid in a pocket or purse. (Of course, if it is in a pocket, make sure it doesn't accidentally go in the wash!)

At home, have specific designated spots where you store your aids and try not to deviate from those spots. There are usually only three places I put my hearing aids – in one of two drawers in my bathroom, in the medicine cabinet downstairs, or in a special pocket in my purse. If they aren't there, I panic a bit. It means I took my hearing aids off without paying attention and they could be anywhere. I really try to stay conscious when I take those aids off as to remember where I put them. Not only to easily find them, but that they are not in a location that could expose them to harm. Here is a perfect example of what I mean. One evening I was lying on the sofa watching TV. Closed captioning was on and I did not really need the aids. I wanted to take them off but was too comfortable to get up and put them in one of my designated spots. So I took them off and placed them on the windowsill. The window was open. FORTUNATELY, I remembered to grab them and put them in one of their designated spots before going to bed. But if I had forgotten, rain, or even the morning dew, could damage the aids. And, of course, if I still had that cat that loved earwax, they would be on the floor.

I recommend protecting your investment by acquiring hearing aid insurance. We insure our cars. Our homes. Insure your aids. You do pay a deductible, but it is MUCH less expensive than paying another several thousand to replace a hearing aid or two.

In conclusion:

Hearing aids are devices designed to assist those with imperfect hearing. They do not restore one to perfect hearing. They are often imperfect, expensive and bothersome devices; they are small, fragile, and require your care. Having and wearing them is a far better alternative than the negative consequences of not wearing them. There are additional devices and technologies that can help you with your hearing loss.

Chapter 7 References and Resources:

Oticon. (2014). *Oticon Product Showcase.* Retrieved January 2014, from Oticon: http://www.oticonusa.com/product-showcase.aspx

Associates, Audiology. (n.d).. *Our Staff.* Retrieved January 2014, from Audiology Associates: http://www.audiologyassociates.net/audiologists-santa-clarita-ca

Reports, C. (2013). *Hearing Aid Buyers Guide.* Retrieved from Consumer Reports: http://www.consumerreports.org/cro/hearing-aids/buying-guide.htm

RERC. (n.d).. *Dr. Ross on Hearing Loss.* Retrieved from Rehabilitation Engineering Research Center on Hearing Enhancement: http://hearingresearch.org/ross/index.php

Phonak. (n.d).. *The Forums.* Retrieved June 2014, from Hearing Like Me: http://www.hearinglikeme.com/

Etsy. (2014). *Echoings.* Retrieved June 17, 2014, from Etsy.com: https://www.etsy.com/shop/Echoings

Linnaea Mallette

CHAPTER 8:
ADDITIONAL ASSISTIVE DEVICES AND TECHNOLOGY

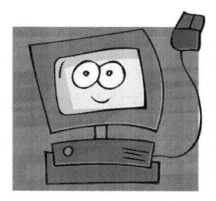

Besides hearing aids, which earned their own chapter[9], other technologies and devices are helpful when getting along in the world with a hearing loss. What I am sharing here is from my own personal experience. There are many other devices and technologies available that I haven't utilized and likely do not know about.

Bluetooth-based devices

Personalized Sound Amplification

With Bluetooth technology, we are seeing the advent of user-programmable hearing devices coming on the market. They are not designed for individuals with a severe loss, and the jury is still out on just how effective they really are, but this technology is in its infancy and will surely become more sophisticated. I invite you to read a particular article on the New York Times site titled, "Better Hearing Through Bluetooth". Read many of the comments to the article too. There are readers who have successfully purchased aids online at considerable savings after submitting a hearing test.

It pays to do research!

---

[9] See Chapter: Hearing Aids – Saving Grace – Necessary Evil

Assistance for Communication

Email

Email is the best. Why? Because no hearing is required. No lip reading. Everything is written out. It does have its limitations, though, on discussions that are long and complex. When it comes to email, I follow the guidance given to me by one of my bosses years ago, *"if a situation isn't resolved in 2 emails, I pick up the phone..."*

The Cell Phone – Especially a Smartphone

I think Smartphones are the best invention since computers. They serve us all so well in a myriad of ways – especially if we are hearing impaired.

I Access Email from my cell phone.

Text messaging. "Texting" as it is commonly called, is a form of email, but done via a phone network, not a computer or web network. Not great for long messages, but certainly great for quick important information like times, places (addresses), 'yes' or 'no' simple communication and conveying of critical information.

Notes: There is another surprising way to use text messaging without actually "sending" the message: using the text feature when the environment requires whispering (or when in an environment where it is so loud you cannot hear..).. A thoughtful professional used his cell phone's text features for communication with me. This is what happened:

I was at a conference videotaping. One of the keynote speakers had his own film crew there videotaping as well. The person they were videotaping was the first of three speakers, so they could not go up and dismantle their equipment until all three speakers were finished talking.

I was taping the second speaker when one of the film crewmembers came up and tried to whisper something in my left ear. I firmly whispered I could not hear him. He walked to the other ear and tried to whisper....I shooed him away shouting in a whisper that I was half-deaf and couldn't hear him. He would have to write the message if he wanted me to get it.

He came back a couple minutes later with his cell phone and the text, "I left the light on for you."

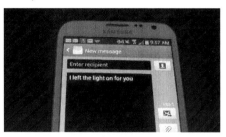

He did not send the text; he opened a new text message, typed what he was trying to tell me and walked over to show me. I was SO moved by this gesture. Not only because he was leaving his professional lights on for my videotaping, but that he made the effort to communicate that to me. He didn't just shrug his shoulders and give up. I was so appreciative I almost welled up in tears.

I was grateful, once again, for the convenience technology, like computers and cell phones, offers to those of us with imperfect hearing and those who are trying to communicate with us. You might consider this when persons with a hearing loss just are not catching what you are saying or you notice they are not connected to the conversation at hand. Using your text or note feature on your cell phone, draft a message, show it to them and enable them to participate, to connect.

Of course, pen and paper work well too.

Skype®

I rely heavily on Skype to keep in touch with my friend and business partner Circe Denyer. Skype! (Now a Microsoft product) enables me to communicate with Circe by instant messaging via the computer using text and video. The video is used rarely, but when I need it, it's a lifesaver. I use it when we are collaborating on a project and it is time consuming and awkward to text back and forth. With a headset and video, it is as if she's right there in the room, FACING ME, so I have the benefit of reading her face, eyes and lips as we are working. In the near future, we will be conducting training and meetings via Skype, where up to 10 people can participate and ALL of their faces can show IF they all use webcams.

There are numerous other features Skype offers – some free, some not. Hearing impaired or not, it is a worthwhile service to use. The services I use are free. Below is a snapshot of our chat window for instant texting:

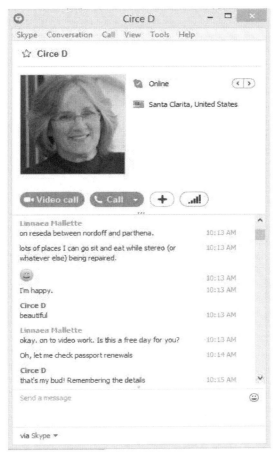

Assistance for USING the Phone

Talking on the Phone:

People who know me know I would prefer not to talk on the phone. Sometimes there is no getting around it and I must. If the phone connection is bad, I'll pull my husband in to listen for me. Often times when the person on the other end realizes how much trouble I am having, they will offer to send me an email instead.

When I am calling businesses, I explain right from the beginning, "I am hard of hearing. If you will speak just a little bit louder and slower I usually do all right." IF I just say, "I am hard of hearing" they have this button to crank up the volume. Well, cranking up the volume doesn't usually work. I need clarity too!

If I get someone with a strong accent, I will ask if there is someone else I can talk to. If not, I ask someone to hear for me via a conference call or to simply listen and relay what is being said to me. Sort of like an interpreter. I may also hang up and call back using a voice transcription service (more on that coming up.).

Telecoils

A feature available on many hearing aids, "telecoil" is also referred to as a "t-switch" or "t-coil." I personally have never enjoyed using the telecoil feature on my aids. It requires holding the phone in a strange fashion that is unnatural and uncomfortable for me. I can never seem to get the earpiece on the phone lined up right with the microphone on my hearing aid. I usually end up taking my hearing aid off, or using the streamer (see below). The problem with removing one's aid, however, is losing it! When I DO exercise patience and use the telecoil feature on my aids (previously the 4th switch on the hearing aid), the ability to hear better on the phone is improved.

Streamers and Other Bluetooth Devices

Bluetooth technology (the "streamer" for example) essentially turns hearing aids into wireless headsets. I do have a streamer, which again, I do not use very much because it requires more wires to manage, more things to charge, more stuff hanging off my physical body and wearing hearing aids longer than I'm comfortable. BUT, when I do use the streamer for phone calls, music computer or TV, the clarity is remarkable.

Made for IPhone Hearing Aids

The newest technology that has come out in April of 2014 is "Made for iPhone hearing aids." Three manufacturers have released this technology, and all are a little different. Some hearing aids can now be connected directly to an iPhone eliminating the need for a streamer. Others can use the streamer, allowing for adjustments to the hearing aids using the iPhone. Plans for Android phones to connect to hearing aids are in the works.

Microphones and FM systems

Many hearing aids can be connected to an external microphone that will help the hearing aid user hear the speaker as if they are wearing headphones. Some of these connect through a streamer, or through a connecter worn on the hearing aid. Children in school often use the FM version using a part clipped on to the hearing aid. The microphone would also be helpful in meeting situations.

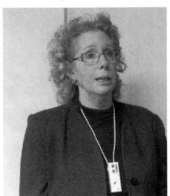

Oticon, which is the brand of hearing aids I own, has created what is called a "ConnectLine Microphone." It is a discreet microphone that a person clips on and connects wirelessly to the streamer. When the person wearing the microphone speaks, his/her voice goes right into the hearing aids.

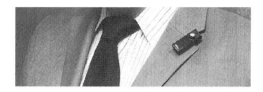

The clarity is remarkable. A person can stand as far as 16 yards from me and it still works. This is very useful when chatting in the car as it can eliminate the need to be face to face, thus minimizing the danger of driving with a hearing loss[10]. This is another technology I've not utilized much, BUT when I once complained to my audiologist about an especially difficult time I had hearing a lady sitting across from me while dining outside, she suggested that in the future I have my little ConnectLine microphone with me and hand it to the other person. Given THAT, I just might take advantage of this little device.

Google® Voice

I rely on Google Voice to help deliver messages from callers, transcribed to text and emailed to me. I do not use many features. What I do use is so helpful.

This is how it works for me:

A person calls and I do not answer the phone. It goes to voice mail.

The recorded voice mail says something like, "You've reached Linnaea Mallette. Please leave a message and it will be transcribed for her to retrieve."

These transcribed messages are emailed to me. I simply open the email and read the transcription. The email always includes a link to the voice mail itself so I can listen to it or save it.

If the person talked too long or too inaudibly, the email will say it was unable to transcribe the message but still provides a link so I can listen to the voice mail myself.

The transcription is not perfect, but it is usually enough for me to figure out what the message is. Below is an example of what Google Voice did with a message. For privacy reasons the phone number is not

---

[10] See Chapter: Dangers of Hearing Loss

included, but it was in the original transcription. I have bolded the word corrections. The grammatical errors are obvious.

Google Voice Version:

"Hello Mallette, This is at net. McCollough with house master. I'm calling on the subject. I'm judging. I do have a phone battery of judges for the September the 7th contest. And I was calling you about your availability. To judge another contact on Wednesday evening September, the 18th. This is area of the 21 and 23. And it's Elizabeth cartons, area, so if you could let me know, that would be great. I'm at (XXX) XXX-XXXX. Thanks."

What was actually said:

"Hello Mallette. This is **Annette McCollough** with **Toastmasters.** I'm calling on the subject **of** judging. I do have a **full** battery of judges for the September 7th contest. And I was calling you about your availability to judge another **contest** on Wednesday evening, September the 18th. This is Area 21 and 23. And it's Elizabeth **Carder's area,** so if you could let me know that would be great. I'm at (XXX) XXX-XXXX. Thanks"

So, Google Voice is an imperfect science, but it is a perfect solution to those of us who do not hear well on the phone. It gives us a good heads up on what the call is about.

Captioned Telephones

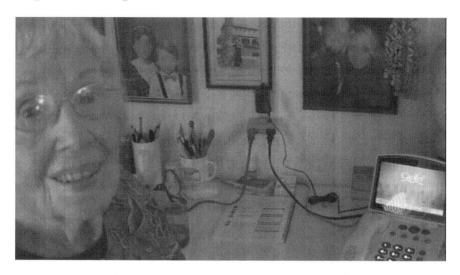

A captioned telephone is a special telephone that has a built-in screen to display everything a caller says as text. A captioned phone connects to both your phone service and the internet. The internet connects to a Captioned Telephone Service (CTS) that, by use of voice recognition technology, transcribes conversations that then show up as captions on the phone's screen.

The lovely woman pictured above is Marylou Denyer. She recently acquired a CapTel telephone. With the CapTel phone, a person is transcribing what the caller is saying. They are not privy to what you, the CapTel owner, is saying. Consequently, the captioned results are far more accurate than Google Voice.

I did a video interview with Marylou and her daughter, Circe Denyer, who happens to be a PC technician. The video is about 12 minutes long and you can hear what the experience was like for Marylou. The video includes a live demonstration of what an incoming call looks like on the phone.

The ease and reliability of the captioning does depend on the type of internet service you have. While the CapTel installation specialist and the customer service people are very helpful and knowledgeable, they will not come out to troubleshoot problems with the phone after they have installed it. You would have to rely on a technician or your internet service provider, depending on the source of the problem, to help you troubleshoot the captioning.

If you have a high-speed cable connection, you will have far less challenges than if you have a connection via a phone line, a DSL connection. DSL is what Marylou has. If the connection is not clear and strong, the captions may not work.

There are two primary problems and solutions when the captions are not working on a CapTel phone with DSL internet connection:

DSL Filter

Telephones make noise on the same line the computer uses. A DSL filter is required because it filters out the noise so the computer can have a clear channel to exchange data between the computer and the internet server. They can go bad, so it is important to make sure the filter is new.

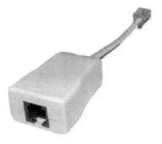

DNS settings in the router

If you have any technical knowledge, or know someone who does, change the DNS setting in the router. DNS is the process that translates, for example, "google.com" into to the physical numerical address of that web site. The name, "Google.com" is not what is communicated to the Internet – it is a series of numbers and those numbers are translated into what you see. Using a Google DNS setting of 8.8.8.8 gives your system better translating performance.

CapTel via Digital Phones

It is my understanding, after chatting with a CapTel representative at a recent event, this service works with a digital phone service too. He specifically mentioned Magic Jack. I did some research (since I no longer have a landline) on how reliable the digital phone service is with closed-captioned telephones. It seems that depending, again, on how fast the internet service is, the time it takes for the captioned text to appear on the screen can vary. The most responsive results are via a landline or with high-speed internet.

Many states have CTS and captioned phones available at a reduced price or for no charge to individuals with documented hearing loss. One of the most well-known captioned telephone service providers is CapTel.

Phone Captioning via Smartphones

I was thrilled to discover a service called Hamilton CapTel has an app for Smartphones, which enables you to read what the person you are talking to is saying. Like CapTel, there is an individual transcribing what the caller says – but via your Smartphone.

Much to my surprise, it is free, and no documentation from an audiologist is required to use the service. However, it is a Federal crime to use the service if you do not have a hearing loss. I would guess that the individuals who do the transcribing could determine if the person using the service really has a hearing loss.

You register with the service and receive a designated phone number. Once you download the app to your phone, the captioning service is then available. I did this for my own phone and I found, as with all new technology, it takes some getting used to. The retrieval of text voicemail messages is a bit complicated. The alternative of not understanding calls or voice mail messages makes the learning curve worthwhile.

Next is a screen shot of the captioning coming in on my Smartphone. The person I was speaking with was instructing me how to take a screenshot of the captioning on the phone so I could include it in a blog (and this book).

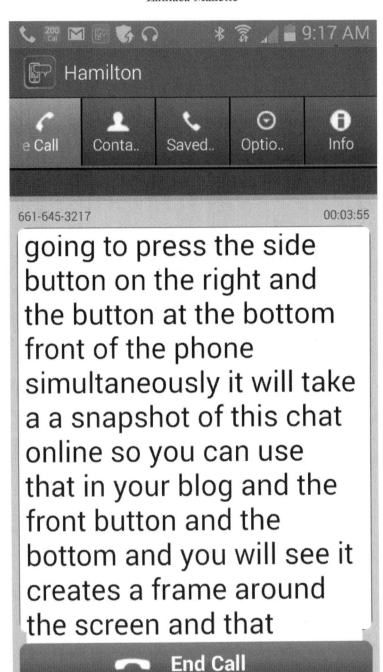

going to press the side button on the right and the button at the bottom front of the phone simultaneously it will take a a snapshot of this chat online so you can use that in your blog and the front button and the bottom and you will see it creates a frame around the screen and that

Assistance for the TV

As stated many times in this book, turning the volume up on the TV so loud it is annoying to others is a sure sign one's hearing is going. Fortunately, there is help when it comes to the TV.

TV Ears®

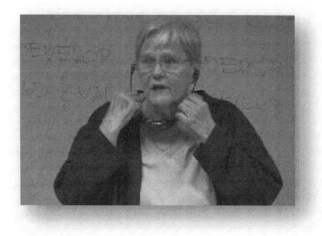

In one of the Toastmaster clubs I belong to is this absolutely delightfully funny member, mentioned earlier, Barbara Massey. She has a natural talent for humor. Whether speaking or just sitting in the audience, she has a sense of humor that doesn't quit. She gave a speech about the fact that as she got older she has lost quite a bit of hearing, and how the TV became a real problem for her.

She didn't get hearing aids right away because they are so expensive. She just played the TV loud. No problem… until she visited her son and family during Christmas one year. It was a family tradition to watch White Christmas. But Barbara could not hear it.

She had heard of wireless headsets and eventually started to walk out of a store with a pair until she noted, printed in very small print on the packaging, that while using the headsets she'd be the only one who could hear the TV. The TV would be silent to anyone else sitting in the room. She was crushed. She wanted to enjoy TV with others.

That is when she discovered TV Ears® through a magazine ad captioned "It Saved Our Marriage!" She purchased them and has enjoyed them for several years. Says Barbara, "greatest invention since the hearing aid." (Yes, she finally got those too!)

Surprisingly, TV Ears® work in movie theaters and playhouses too! Said Barbara about another visit with her son...

"...when we went to the new 007 movie I took just the 'ears' part. Worked great. I know, I know. You wonder WHY I'd need a hearing device at a 007 movie. All the explosions, gunshots and noise. **That** I can hear. It's when he whispers sweet nothings to one of the Bond girls ...THAT'S when they come in real handy!! I don't miss a thing." Fortunately, she allowed her talk to be posted on YouTube.

Closed Captioning

I will never forget the first time I experienced closed captioning on a movie. I was at Harrah's hotel in Las Vegas. I was invited to be a showcase speaker for a Toastmasters Regional conference. This was June 2005. Full scale closed captioning was initiated in 1980. Yes, I was way behind in availing myself of this technology. This was due, in large part, to my not fully embracing or accepting my hearing loss, thus not researching ways to make life easier for me.

One of the two friends who accompanied me to that conference set the captioning to play automatically on the TV in our hotel room. The movie I watched for the first time with closed captioning was "Dumb and Dumber" I nearly died laughing. And at the same time I wanted to cry. I had *no* idea what I had been missing all these years.

Since then I've come to know that closed captioning is not just for those of us with a hearing loss. Closed captioning is for everyone — everyone who doesn't want to miss a word in a movie, that is.

Shortly after my Las Vegas experience, we acquired a closed-captioning device for our TV at home. At that point, TV manufacturers were not mandated to include closed-captioning decoders, and our TV did not have that capability. But there were devices that made it possible, and that's what we got.

At first, the script showing up on the TV was extremely annoying and distracting for my husband. But before long not only did it not annoy him, he enjoyed it, as he himself did not realize how much dialog was inaudible on TV. He just loves not missing a word.

Just the other night we were watching a series called "The Killing." Someone on the show had received a phone call. What was being spoken on the other end of the receiver was being spelled out on the screen. Bruce turned to me and said, "Wow, without this captioning, even I would not be able to hear what is being said through that phone." With the popular show called "Downton Abbey" it would have been hard for both my husband and me to understand those English accents without closed captioning!

Of course, the other benefit of closed captioning is when you cannot enjoy having the volume cranked up – or on at all. Maybe you have touchy neighbors who don't like hearing your TV. Or you have family members trying to sleep. Or it is just plain late and you want to observe the 10:00 PM city ordinance for noise – you can still enjoy the show thanks to closed captioning.

I so appreciate closed captioning that I have started to caption videos of my talks. I just completed my first one, and it came out pretty darn good! That effort was inspired by the recent contact with a woman who has to have captioning to understand anything on YouTube. She was interested in hearing me speak, so I decided it was time to get serious and add captioning to my videos. You can see captioning added to my humorous talk "Front Row Please" — which discusses some of the benefits of hearing loss.

Closed Captioning on Netflix®:

Since Netflix is the rage these days, I must mention it as it relates to closed captioning. We discovered in late 2013 that Netflix had made a large number of the movies available with closed captioning. The closed captioning, however, is carried through the technology of the device that delivers the movie from Netflix. The solution seemed simple enough until you realize that the Blu-Ray® manufacturers do not explicitly mention closed captioning for live streaming, the method of delivery for Netflix movies; anywhere. Not on the boxes. Not on specifications on the web. And for Panasonic® at least, not on their detailed PDF booklet about the product.

Don't count on the folks at the retail stores to know what they are talking about either. Even "experts" at Netflix didn't fully know what we were asking for, or what they were talking about. The people who know whether a device delivers closed captioning for live streaming DO NOT WORK at the stores that sell the players. My husband spent a huge amount of his time reading online to find the brand and model that did send closed captioning to the TV for Netflix movies. Sounds like we were on the right track, right? NOT! When we got to the store, those "oh-so-helpfuls" behind the counter did not assure him that it would work! The discussions went on for 90 minutes. I settled into one of the overstuffed chairs in front of a demo TV and fell asleep.

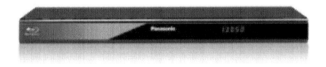

In the end, it worked out because my husband took the plunge, knowing he might have to return the player and try again. The player does in fact deliver a quality, closed caption for many movies on the Netflix Live Stream list and plays 3-D movies to boot. Since the models are being upgraded all the time, just look for a Panasonic® (which is what we have) Blu-Ray player that has integrated Wi-Fi, 3-D and you should be okay.

Alerting Devices

Alerting devices come in all shapes, sizes, and features to alert one with imperfect hearing that something is happening that they probably want to be made aware of. Like an incoming phone call. An alarm clock going off. A doorbell ringing. When one's baby is crying. When a fire or carbon monoxide alarm is triggered. Cell phones (Smartphones) can usually be set to flash a strobe when the phone rings or it gets a text message.

The alerts can be lights flashing, extremely loud noises like horns, or a gentle shaking. Some devices for monitoring babies can analyze and report if the baby sounds hungry, sleepy or bored.

Isn't that remarkable?

I have used various alerting devices – like a light blinking when I had a landline phone, a sonic alarm that "boomed" when it was time to wake up, etc. It startled the hell out of my husband and cats so I had to cease using one. At home, I use the radio setting on an alarm clock. Loud music begins to play and it does wake me up. I use the vibration setting on my phone, which I can hear rattling on a table when not attached to my body.

Hearing Dogs

A good friend's sister-in-law has used hearing dogs for years to help her get along at home. The dogs are trained to make physical contact and lead the hearing-impaired person to the source of the sound. Pretty remarkable. There are hearing dogs that can assist in public as well.

In conclusion:

There are numerous assistive devices and technologies a person with a hearing loss can utilize. The cost, convenience and comfort (for me and those around me), determine the extent to which I avail myself of the assistance.

Chapter 8 References and Resources:

Romano, T. (2014, January 15). *Well*. Retrieved June 15, 2014, from New York Times: http://well.blogs.nytimes.com/2014/01/15/better-hearing-through-bluetooth/?_php=true&_type=blogs&_r=0

Skype: http://www.skype.com/en/

Google voice: The full description of the service is on their site: http://www.google.com/googlevoice/about.html

CapTel video of my interview with Mary Lou Denyer and her daughter: http://youtu.be/ZA7DEpq09MM

Magic Jack internet phone: http://Magicjack.com

Smartphone Captioning App: Hamilton CapTel:
http://www.hamiltoncaptel.com/

Video of talk given by Barbara Massey about her hearing loss and challenges with the TV

http://www.youtube.com/watch?v=QXEmsEs8bHM&feature=youtu.be

CHAPTER 9:
WHAT IS IT LIKE TO LIVE WITH A HEARING LOSS?

"I am just as deaf as I am blind. The problems of deafness are deeper and more complex, if not more important than those of blindness. Deafness is a much worse misfortune. For it means the loss of the most vital stimulus-- the sound of the voice that brings language, sets thoughts astir, and keeps us in the intellectual company of man. Blindness separates us from things but deafness separates us from people" – Helen Keller

The American Speech-Language-Hearing Association (ASHA) explains that hearing loss is measured far beyond decibels. The impact of hearing loss depends on the individual, but overall, hearing loss is linked to feelings of anxiety, frustration, social isolation and fatigue.

I can testify to all of those feelings and experiences.

Why Seeking Help is Important

It is pretty easy to realize someone we know no longer has perfect hearing. But, for the individual with the loss, it may go undetected for years. On an average, a person waits 7-10 years before seeking help. There have been numerous studies done on the impact of hearing loss, as we grow older. The results are startling. Studies have shown that hearing loss can increase the risk of developing dementia.

In 1999, the National Council on Aging conducted a study and prepared a report titled "The Consequences of Untreated Hearing Loss in Older Persons"

The goal of the study was to assess the impact on one's quality of life comparing those wearing hearing aids and those not.

Results Not Wearing Hearing Aids

The report indicated that elderly people in the study who did not wear hearing aids experienced many negative mental and emotional consequences like sadness, depression, anxiety, isolation, insecurity, and paranoia. These results were the same regardless of gender, age, and income.

Results Wearing Hearing Aids

The results were quite different for those elderly folks who did wear hearing aids. A significant improvement on the overall quality of their life and the lives of those they live with was reported. Over half reported better relationships with family and friends. They could interact better with their grandchildren. They experienced increased confidence and a sense of independence.

What Hearing Loss Feels Like

A colleague at work, having just returned from being out due to a serious head cold, told me she didn't know how I got along as well as I do. She found the inability to hear clearly was not only excruciatingly frustrating, but also she felt alienated and lonely. "I cannot imagine living my life that way."

If I had to sum up the experience of hearing loss in just one word, it would be "frustrating." No matter when or how the loss occurs — at an early age or later in life — the inability to hear speech and many of the sounds of everyday life is frustrating. It is frustrating not only for the one with the loss, but for those around him/her as well. Dr. Ross nailed it when he said, – "When someone in the family has a hearing loss, the whole family has a hearing problem." It is SO true. I extend that hearing problem way beyond the family unit. The workplace; the marketplace; the place of worship; any place where the participation of a person is important for action or satisfaction. That is every place.

In a wonderful resource called "Facing the Challenge – a Survivor's Manual for the Hard of Hearing People" compiled by the Hearing Loss Association of Oregon, a woman shares her experience as a person with a hearing loss. The discourse is called "Frustrations and other Emotions" by Karen Swezey.

I have taken some of the key points of her sharing and presented them in **bold** followed by my own personal experiences.

Hearing loss is difficult. Largely because communication is difficult. It is also difficult because I must take extra precautions when walking, cooking, driving or doing a number of simple life tasks. I have to make sure I'm not missing something that could cause property or personal damage.

Lots of emotions. Emotions like anger, humiliation, frustration, are a common experience, even when I am up front about a hearing loss. I'm getting better at avoiding overreacting when in a negative hearing situation. However, it does depend on the importance of the interaction and my state of mind/confidence at that moment.

It is tiring. When I can, I take a nap every day at mid-day. It takes an enormous amount of emotional, psychological and physical energy to strain to hear what I can and "read" and interpret everything else. It is exhausting. When I worked at UCLA, I used to literally grab a pillow and lie down on the floor to rest in between sessions of teaching. Co-workers found it amusing; for me, it was survival.

Challenges to our self-esteem. When people show impatience with my limitation, it feels awful and wears on my self-csteem. This is why I chose to hide my hearing loss for a good part of my life. I couldn't stand the pain of "rejection." As stated in the beginning of the book about when I skydived, I was willing to face death than the pain associated with the instructor and fellow skydiver's reactions to my hearing loss.

Decisions made without asking us first. This can happen when going to a public event. I'm often able to sit up close. There have been occasions where instead of sitting me up close at an event, they sit me next to a huge TV screen in the back of the room. That is like watching TV with no closed captioning. Useless.

Many factors affect our ability to hear. For me, it can be the way a person speaks. Does he have an accent? Does she mumble? Is he even facing me? Does he have a habit of putting his hands in front of his mouth when speaking (a sign of insecurity or uncertainty). If he has a mustache or bucked teeth, I'm in trouble. If a person is wearing dentures that are not secured and flap when he talks it is like seeing double. I cannot read the lips.

Background noise is a problem too. Is there background noise going on that competes with my ability to hear? In some cases, that background noise can be reduced. Toastmaster clubs that meet in restaurants often are able to have the music in the adjacent meeting room turned down or off. I recently asked a car dealership to turn down the music in the display room so I could better hear what the salesperson was saying to me. Some comply willingly, some don't (or can't). Unfortunately, there is usually no option with background noise except to hope one of my hearing aid settings successfully minimizes the impact on my hearing. If not, I may just remove my aids altogether.

Some days we are stronger than others. On the days when I am not as strong – physically or emotionally –as other days, I just don't hear as well. I may refrain from fully participating or postpone doing activities I am obligated to do because of the increased difficulty in hearing and my reaction to the associated challenges accentuated.

There are always people who just do not get it and don't make any effort to help us hear. Those people I pretty much avoid, or I ask a friend to accompany me and I ask that person to translate for me.

I have heard this from other folks who have hearing loss. I am not alone.

What Hearing Loss Sounds Like

The cover image for book titled, "Shouting Won't Help", by Katherine Bouton is of a woman with her head submerged under water just up over her ears. Have you ever been in a swimming pool or bathtub where your head was submerged and someone was trying to talk to you? It is impossible to understand what is being said. Speech is just chunks of sound; there are resources to HEAR what it sounds like to not hear.

For example, the House Research Institute created a wonderful video that really opens one's eyes as to what hearing loss sounds like. They took a Flintstones cartoon and adjusted the audio to remove the range of sounds a person with mild-moderate-and severe loss would not hear. Of course, having a significant loss, all the examples sound pretty much the same to me. My husband watched the video and, for the first time in our nearly three decades of marriage, he better understands what I'm dealing with. Google "Fred Flintstone Hearing Loss" and you will find several places where it is housed on YouTube.

Starkey has a hearing loss simulator you can use on line. A truly comprehensive simulator is from the Office of Mine Safety and Health Research. It is available as a download or one can purchase the CD.

Environmental Sounds I Don't Hear

Here is a list of what I cannot hear in my environment; it is by NO means all-inclusive:

> **Birds** – The everyday birds that grace our trees. If you put on a recording of a bird aviary, it is a recording of silence for me. I do hear crows and seagulls.
>
> **Crickets.**
>
> **Buzzers** – Many, many of the buzzes of timers, alarm clocks, cell phone rings. I respond better to foghorns and cowbells. I used to have a "sonic boom" alarm clock that would send my cats and husband fleeing from the bed like a speeding bullet.
>
> **Rain** – I often am shocked when I open the door to head out and realize it is raining!
>
> **Glass breaking** – I add this because during the earthquake of 1994 (we were 4 miles from epicenter) we had many glass items break, but I did not hear them and was shocked when I went downstairs and saw the amount of damage the earthquake inflicted that I did not hear. Fortunately, I was wearing shoes and did not get cut.
>
> **Sirens** – I do not hear sirens until they are almost on top of me.
>
> **Whispering** – no matter how "loud" a person whispers.
>
> **Water running.**

My left ear is worse. I hear normally for just a few decibels, and then it drops like a jagged cliff from there.

Speech Sounds I Don't Hear

In speech, I do not hear 'c', 's', 'ch', 'sh', 't'

For those who like visual imagery, here is a somewhat crude visual representation of what I cannot hear, environmentally and in speech.

LOSS IN MY LEFT EAR

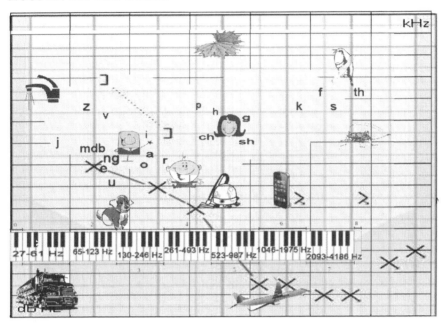

LOSS IN MY RIGHT EAR

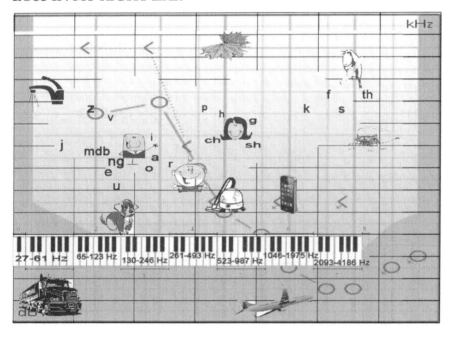

Sounds shown above the markers are those I cannot hear. Note the decibel range of the octaves of the piano. I do not hear the last octave of a piano – whether I am wearing hearing aids or not. Some sounds I hear by themselves, but become obscure if competing with other noise. Take the vacuum cleaner. Vacuum cleaners are mighty loud. But if I am listening to something else at the same time, (music, TV) the sound of the vacuum cleaner is diffused, for lack of a better word, and I'm not always positive what the sound is I'm hearing.

Here is a perfect example of what I'm talking about. We live in a townhome complex two doors down from a pair of Chihuahuas. These little guys punch huge volume for their little bodies. If these pups are barking on the patio while we are watching TV, my husband has to turn off the TV until the dogs stop barking because he can't hear the TV.

Not me!

With the TV on, I don't even hear the dogs barking. "Boy, that is sure a benefit of not hearing well," my husband often remarks. True. There are some benefits. More about those in the next chapter.

Speech Comes in Chunks

Speech comes at me in chunks, sounding very much like having a head cold or having ears submerged in water. I translate those chunks of sound into something I can understand by knowing the topic, and/or the personality of the speaker. Often my husband will blow his nose (or emit other bodily function noises) and I'd poke my head in and ask, "What honey?" But it gets much more complicated than that...

The words, "sign on the door" sounds to me like "I –N-OR"; so, if my husband says that from downstairs, and I'm in a good mood, I might hear, "I adore," or "I'm game for," or something playful like that. If, on the other hand, I'm in a bad mood, I might hear, "I ignore," or "I don't care," or "I snore," or any combination of annoying words. If I know he's talking about expecting someone to come by that day, I will figure out that he has said something about putting a sign on the door. A good 50% of my hearing is done this way. Most of it I do almost unconsciously, but it is tiring. I usually don't have problems falling asleep – especially since it isn't noise that would keep me awake!

You may ask, after reading this, how it is I am able to hear and communicate. You'll learn more about that in the Dynamics of Hearing[11]. But for now I will confess that I also bluff. I bluff a lot.

In conclusion:

Hearing loss affects what people can hear in their environment, their degree of connection with others, and sense of well-being and happiness, which varies from day to day.

---

[11] See Chapter: Dynamics of Hearing

Chapter 9 References and Resources:

Bouton, K. (2013). Shouting Won't Help - Why I - and 50 Million Other Americans - Can't Hear You. New York: Sarah Crichton Books.

Romano, T. (2014, January 15). *Well*. Retrieved June 15, 2014, from New York Times: http://well.blogs.nytimes.com/2014/01/15/better-hearing-through-bluetooth/?_php=true&_type=blogs&_r=0

NCOA. (1999). *The Consequences of Untreated Hearing Loss in Older Persons*. Washington DC: National Council on the Aging.

NCOA. (1999). *The Impact of Hearing Loss on Quality of LIfe in Older Adults*. Washington DC: The Gerontological Society of America.

HHH, Oregon. (n.d).. *Facing the Challenge -0 A Survivor's Manual for Hard of Hearing People*. Retrieved December 2013, from Hearing Loss Association of America Kentucky Chapter: http://www.hearinglossky.org/hlasurvival1.html

Starky hearing loss stimulator: http://www.starkey.com/hearing-loss-simulator

Office of Mine Safety and Health Research Comprehensive hearing loss simulator: http://www.cdc.gov/niosh/mining/works/coversheet1820.html

Skype: http://www.skype.com/en/

Google voice: The full description of the service is on their site: http://www.google.com/googlevoice/about.html

Video of my interview with Mary Lou Denyer and her daughter: http://youtu.be/ZA7DEpq09MM

Magic Jack internet phone: http://Magicjack.com

Smartphone Captioning App: Hamilton Captel: http://www.hamiltoncaptel.com/

Video of talk given by Barbara Massey about her hearing loss and challenges with the TV

http://www.youtube.com/watch?v=QXEmsEs8bHM&feature=youtu.be

Linnaea's humorous talk "Front Row Please" — which discusses some of the benefits of hearing loss.

https://www.youtube.com/watch?v=8iu1jXFFdQY&feature=youtu.be

CHAPTER 10:
BENEFITS OF HEARING LOSS

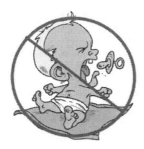

While the disadvantages far outweigh the advantages of having a hearing loss, there are a few benefits worth mentioning. I already mentioned in the previous chapter how annoying sounds are often washed out in the face of competing sounds. Here are some more advantages:

Arguments

I have to confess, I only use this tactic on my husband. As we grow old together, the need to employ it is less and less. If my husband is on a nagging fit or seemingly unreasonable, I turn off my aids and turn my back. That discussion is over!

Avoiding Undesirable Requests

I think this is a form of "selective hearing." Sometimes, when younger and more rebellious, I'd feign not hearing a request to refrain from doing something I didn't want to do. When questioned later why something wasn't done, I'd innocently respond, "Oh, must have misunderstood what you said."

Eavesdropping

On occasion, I "eavesdrop" in my own fashion, utilizing the dynamics of hearing[12] that I am especially skilled at. I rarely catch an entire conversation, but with snatches of the lips combined with facial and

---

[12] See Chapter: Dynamics of Hearing

body language, I can surmise pretty well the essence of a conversation going on from across the room.

Babysitting

Depending on how you feel about babysitting those younger relatives – nieces, nephews, and grandchildren – the fact that they are hard to understand is a legitimate excuse not to babysit. For example, when my nieces were five and two, if the older niece came to me crying because something has happened to the younger niece, it would be important to understand what she is saying. I cannot understand the chatter of young children.

Noise Pollution

For me, the biggest benefit is the control of noise pollution. Each day I waited for the bus to UCLA I was grateful for the ability to turn off my aids and soften the deafening roar of rush hour traffic.

Public Transit

If I had my druthers, I'd prefer to have a seat all to myself when using public transportation, whether a bus, train or even an airplane.

I have found if I sit on the bus, for example, with my hearing aids fully exposed, the seat next to me is usually left empty unless the bus is nearly full. In that event, the person who does take the seat does not strike up small talk. I may not always enjoy a seat to myself, but I can enjoy a quiet ride.

But sometimes this fails in a big way.

When I traveled to Vermont to meet my future husband's family, I chose to tour the country by train, using Vermont as one of the stops. I employed my technique of exposing my hearing aids, and it worked pretty well. During one leg of the train trip it really backfired on me. An extremely handsome young man bent over, cleared his throat and asked, "Excuse me, is this seat available?" I immediately pulled my hair over my ears to hide the aids and smiled sweetly, "Why yes, it is!" motioning him to sit down. He promptly went and retrieved his grandfather –a tall, unkempt, un-bathed man with sandals sporting dirty toenails! That isn't what I had in mind!

On airplanes, unless we purchase an extra seat, we are going to have someone sitting next to us. But, with hearing aids exposed, I can keep that mindless chatter to a minimum. If there is a fussy baby or noisy child on the plane, I can reach up, click off the aids, and enjoy the quiet.

Front Row Seats

Most event coordinators make provisions for those of us with imperfect hearing by having reserved seating close to the front of an event. Need I expand on how wonderful THIS opportunity is? Now, I don't always need to sit close. Depending on the acoustics of the room, the quality of the microphone, and the way a speaker talks, I can sit in the back of a room and do quite well (once I know the content of a conversation, of course). I often ask to sit closer because the experience is just more intimate when you can see the whites of the presenter's eyes.

But, this doesn't always work out the way I want it to, either!

When the then-President Clinton visited UCLA, I wanted to bypass the thongs of crowds, lines and security by using my hearing loss to secure a seat up close. I mean, I wanted to be up close and personal with Mr. Clinton. (Um, well, not THAT personal!)

So, I pulled my hair back so the aids were clearly visible. I added a limp to my walk, and bypassed the winding lines that made lines at Disneyland look puny, and approached the security men guarding the doors to Pauley Pavilion. With an especially thick "accent" I said, "I need to sit close" pointing to my hearing aids, "I need to read lips." The guard quickly replied, "No problem, we can take care of that." I was doing cartwheels inside...until I was escorted to the very, very top of Pauley Pavilion, joining the pigeons (another species of birds I can hear) right next to a huge projection screen. "There, you can clearly see his lips here," the guard proudly explained, thinking he was doing me a huge favor.

President Clinton was so far away it would have taken binoculars to see his lips. I could have had the same experience sitting at home and watching him on TV. In fact, it would have been better because there would have been captioning on the TV. It is not what I had in mind! TODAY I would have said something. Back then, I was not assertive. Sadly, most of us with a hearing loss are not assertive enough to press for additional help when the initial attempt doesn't meet our needs.

An Ear for Quality

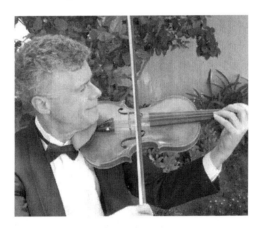

While I do not hear well, I do have an ear for quality. I can listen to classical music and determine the period, and often, the composer. Even more amazing is that if it is a violin solo, I can sometimes identify the soloist by the sound of the violin! I can usually pick out a violin being played by Itzhak Perlman or Anne Sophie Mutter. When my husband (pictured above) is shopping for violins, he actually takes me along! You should see the faces of the sales people when he is sawing away at a violin, asking his hard-of-hearing spouse what she thinks of the way it sounds. If I am naughty I will utter a guttural "good", which embarrasses him, but I find the look on the sales people's faces, well, simply delicious.

In conclusion:

As with every adverse situation or condition, there is some good, some humor that is gleaned from a hearing loss. Use it to your advantage.

CHAPTER 11:
DANGERS OF HEARING LOSS

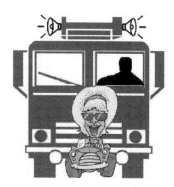

Besides the psychological dangers of hearing loss – especially untreated loss[13] and the dangers of low self-esteem as a result of the loss[14] – there are physical dangers of diminished hearing with everyday living. Note that talking on the phone or listening to an MP3 player compromises your ability to hear and puts you at risk too.

My Experiences:

Parking Lots, Driveways, Intersections

Parking lots, driveways and intersections are a big risk. People backing out or driving forward assume we will hear their cars and move out of the way. Not if our hearing is compromised!

Recently I was walking down the road in a mortuary and a friend pulled me close to the curb to let a car pass by. I did HEAR a noise, but it was so obscured I had not yet figured out it was an oncoming car. Eventually I would have, but in different circumstances, it might have been too late.

When a hearing-impaired person is focused on talking to another — and it does take our entire focus, as we must read lips, face, body language as well as listen — we are distracted from paying attention to

---

[13] See Chapter: Do You Have a Hearing Loss?
[14] See Chapter: My Story

our surroundings. It is wise to alert those around you to watch out for you, just in case. Like my friend who, knowing I was not aware that a car was approaching, pulled me gently over to the side so the car could pass.

Intersections really scare me. I may not hear a car starting to make a right turn while I step off the curb.

Thankfully, car horns are still loud and in the low frequency range. I hear car horns honk. Most people do not honk their car horns through a mortuary, or backing out of parking stalls.

Those trucks that have the beeping noise when backings up (or forklifts in warehouse stores like Costco or Home Depot) are often in the higher frequencies, and if I don't have my aids on, I usually don't hear them.

It is important to pay attention to your surroundings – always. Again, that is hard to do if you are paying attention to a person talking to you. Best to save those parking lot conversations or rants until you are safe in the car (unless you are driving) or at home.

Driving

I did an animated cartoon about driving with a hearing loss titled "Hearing Impaired Grandpa Drives." The gist of the cartoon is that Grandpa has to read lips and turns his head to look at the grandkids in the back seat. Turning his head to look at them in the back seat almost gets them killed. Point? Being the driver and having passengers, as a hearing-impaired person is no laughing matter. IT IS DANGEROUS. Why? Because folks like me, need to read your lips! I cannot watch the road and your lips at the same time!

Oh, I've tried. Many times, I've tried. And it just doesn't work. Looking over to catch pieces of a conversation hoping I can comprehend it, or adjusting my rear view mirror so I can see the lips of passengers in the back seat is begging for an accident. Taking one's attention off the road for just five seconds is enough time to travel the length of a football field. I have nearly sideswiped other drivers or a wall, many times. I most always swerve outside the driving lane. I have learned in my older, wiser years that being polite and doing my best to listen while driving just is not worth risking my life and the life of my passengers.

Whenever possible, if riding with others, I refrain from driving. I even go so far as to have friends and family drive my own car so I can sit in the passenger seat. If circumstances make it necessary for me to drive, I suggest I do most of the talking so we are engaged, catching up on stuff without putting our lives in danger. Once we reach our destination, my passengers can talk their hearts out and have my full attention — on their lips, face, and body.

If you are riding with someone who has a hearing loss, either take the wheel, or be satisfied with listening to the hearing-impaired driver carry the bulk of the conversation, or listening to the radio. Please, please, don't insist on carrying on a conversation that requires the driver to HEAR what you are saying.

If you are riding with a hearing-impaired person who is in denial and you notice that whenever you talk his/her eyes are off the road on you, do the right thing and minimize your side of the conversation. Engage the driver in a conversation by asking questions and letting him/her answer. If all else fails, feign a headache and recline in the seat with your eyes closed.

No if, ands, or buts about it. A hearing-impaired person cannot drive and listen at the same time.

The other danger in driving with your hearing compromised (including talking on the cell phone or blasting the car stereo) is the sound of emergency vehicle sirens. I usually do not hear these until they are right on top of me. What I do is pay attention to traffic patterns. If I see cars suddenly pulling over, I know an emergency vehicle is approaching. If I am behind someone at a red light and it goes green but the person does not go, I no longer just rush around him or her. They might be sitting there because of an approaching fire engine. I was nearly killed twice doing that. Now I WAIT, look around to see what other drivers are doing, before impatiently driving around a person sitting in the vehicle and not moving right away.

The Workplace

The workplace also harbors dangers for those of us with a hearing loss.

I had a scary experience several years ago while still employed at UCLA. It was the afternoon of the final workday before the Christmas holiday break. We were usually released early — like 3:00 or so — on such glorious days. On THIS particular day, I was focused on an e-learning project. I looked up and realized it was very late in the afternoon and VERY quiet.

VERY quiet.

I got up and walked around the suite. It was a ghost town. Everyone was gone. Apparently, the announcement was made that we could leave, and I did not hear it, and no one stopped by to make sure I did.

Scary. Why? What if that announcement was telling us to vacate the building due to a bomb threat or fire? After that experience, I asked the management to make sure that "check on Linnaea" was on the list of things the team leaders must do during an emergency evacuation. I may need to be walking next to someone who will explain what is going on if additional instructions are being given and there are no lips for me to read.

Since then, whenever we had reason to vacate the building, whether for a drill or for real, someone always stopped by to make sure that I was not only aware of the notification, but that I knew WHAT to do as well.

So, public service announcements over a PA system? They do not work for someone like me, a person with imperfect hearing.

Solo Sports

I naturally shy away from sports activities because I do not hear. Imagine being out in left field in a softball game and someone shouts an important piece of information, critical to the game or play, and you don't hear it. Doesn't work. I've done it. Team members get pretty upset.

Nevertheless, it didn't keep me from doing "solo" sports like skydiving experience[15] riding a bike or roller-skating. All are dangerous if no

---

[15] See Chapter: My Story

precautions are taken when hearing is compromised.

Let's take roller-skating. I used to roller-skate a lot around a five-mile parameter of Balboa Park in the San Fernando Valley. That path is shared with bike riders. In addition to not having good hearing, I was (stupidly) listening to loud music too through my headset. I did not hear three bicyclists approaching – didn't hear their bikes, their horns, or their voices, alerting me they were coming up from behind.

Suddenly I was on the ground with two bikes piled up around me. No one was hurt, thankfully, but one of the bicyclists was pretty irritated at me that I didn't heed their warning as they were approaching. How could I? I COULD NOT HEAR THEM!

Today, if I were to go roller-skating I would have someone with me. For a brief period, I thought maybe a T-shirt made that says on the back of it – "Hearing Impaired" would work. But, not if someone wants to sneak up on me and rob or rape me!

I do not do bicycling at all. I cannot hear approaching cars, and I do not hear anyone shouting any warnings to me…it just isn't fun. It's dangerous. I don't go there.

The Kitchen

The kitchen can be dangerous because I do not hear water. I don't hear it running. I don't hear it boiling. When I turn on the water to fill pots and pans, I have to stand there until they are full and then turn off the water. If I dare turn to do something else while the pots and pans are filing. I risk forgetting to turn off the water and it flows onto the floor. Seriously, it is a miracle I have not flooded or burned our place down yet.

Why? I do not hear fire alarms or until just recently, food timers.

It doesn't matter what type of timer it is, I usually do not hear it when it goes off. I find that if I'm engaged in something else, it is enough to cause me not to hear even the best of timers. What I do is set a timer right in front of me when I am at my computer in my home office and watch for it to go off. It vibrates the table a bit, so I usually don't miss it. But it HAS to be right in front of me.

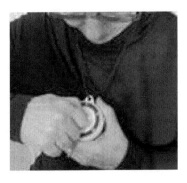

Good news is I just recently discovered and acquired a timer than hangs around my neck. Not only is it loud and long, I FEEL it on my body when it goes off.

Prior to the acquisition of this latest timer, if I missed the timer and forget I have food in the oven, the smoke may trigger the fire alarm, which I don't hear either.

Doctor Visits

Not hearing exactly what the doctor, nurse or pharmacist is saying can be dangerous. Again, the material for a cartoon titled, "The Hearing Impaired Elderly Patient". In the cartoon the elderly patient is all about town with someone half his age living it up. His doctor happens to see him out in public prancing around and questions him about his behavior during his next doctor visit. "I'm just doing what you said at my last physical…" the old man remarks, "Get a hot mama and be cheerful."

The doctor replied in alarm, "No! I said that you had a heart murmur and be careful!"

Funny! However, in real life, it is not a laughing matter.

I recently had to have a minor laser procedure done on each eye. Realizing that if I didn't hear the doctor correctly and moved while the laser was on, or about to be turned on, I could ruin my eyes. I cannot imagine being blind and half-deaf too. I reminded the doctor that I was hearing impaired and would not be able to read her lips while staring at the glowing dot in the machine. I asked her to tell me all that is going to happen and what she may say to me to make sure I don't move at the wrong time. Better yet, what else she can do to alert me besides words. Maybe a tap on the shoulder.

Even though pharmacists tell me all about a prescription I may receive, I still read the label to make sure I heard correctly – like the number of doses or number of times a day to take a dosage. Why? The numbers "1", "9" and "2" and "3" sound very similar to me. I don't want to be taking nine doses when it is only supposed to be one! You get the idea.

Taking Action When Not Fully Hearing an Answer

Was That a Yes?

"Would you like a cup of coffee from Mazzas?" I asked my father-in-law as I headed out the door for my morning walk to my favorite country farm store in Vermont. He answered in a few sentences. I couldn't understand what he was saying, but by reading his body language, facial expressions and listening to his tone of voice, I ASSUMED he said "No."

I was very embarrassed when I returned and looking surprised he said, "Where is my cup of coffee?"

I was reminded that when given a long answer to a simple question I need to ask, "Was that a yes or a no?" By doing this, I protect myself (and others).

If you are interacting with a hearing-impaired individual, answer the question FIRST with a "yes" or "no" and then elaborate.

Can I Pet Your Dog?

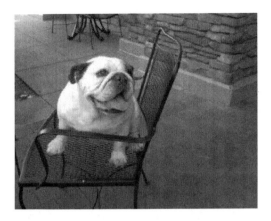

Every week a group of Toastmasters meets for coaching at a local coffee house. There is a group of men who meet there too. But unlike us, they sit outside so a bulldog (named Lola) belonging to one of the men can sit on a chair. Lola sits there as if one of the "guys." For weeks I had wanted to go out and pet that big 'ole bull dog. So one day I went up to the table and asked, "Can I pet your dog? Is she friendly?" The owner responded with a couple of sentences. I wasn't sure what he said, but I studied his body language, facial expressions and listened to his voice. Seemed he was saying it was okay. So I went ahead and petted this big dog. I even put my face up close to the dog's face. Fortunately, that WAS a friendly dog.

But imagine if it wasn't. Imagine the body language, facial expressions and voice tonality was the owners typical response to people to soften his "no" response. I could have had my face bitten off!

So, those of you with imperfect hearing – if you do not get a "yes" or "no" to your question and you don't know what the answer was – ASK. To the dog owner, had I realized how dangerous my assumption could have been, I would have added, "I'm hearing impaired and didn't get all you said, but I think you said it's okay to pet your dog. Yes or no?"

In conclusion:

We place ourselves in dangerous situations when we have a hearing loss, or compromise our hearing by listening to something other than our surroundings or not clarifying if we understood what a person has said.

Chapter 11 References and Resources:

Cartoon: Hearing Loss Grandpa Drives:
https://www.youtube.com/watch?v=M0316-2Osus

Cartoon: "The Hearing Impaired Elderly Patient":
https://www.youtube.com/watch?v=Z4XLvrN1Nvo

CHAPTER 12:
AWKWARD AND DISASTROUS MOMENTS

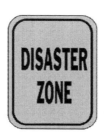

As a person with imperfect hearing, I experience awkward moments almost daily. While it is impossible to control all situations that come our way, it is helpful to be aware of what type of situations could be a source of awkwardness — for you and for those around you. These awkward moments are to help those with a hearing loss and those who are around someone with a hearing loss.

My "Accent"

More times than not, people ask where I am from because I clearly have some sort of accent. They ask something like, "What nationality are you?" I proceed to tell them they are hearing a speech impediment because I have a hearing loss. Hearing that, THEY become stiff, act awkward— and then I feel awkward and the whole interaction is icky. I just had this happen during a Thanksgiving dinner. Lately, what I've been adding to my confession is that I am also a professional speaker, and that I joke with audiences telling them I sound the way I do because I'm from Germany. That usually breaks the discomfort with the person who has asked (and puts my audiences at ease too).

Talking Too Loud

It is difficult to hear the volume of your own voice when wearing hearing aids. When I am in a restaurant, with the din of the noise deafening me even further, I have had friends or family tell me I don't need to be yelling. Usually when THAT happens, I look around the restaurant or party and people are staring at me. Embarrassing.

Humor

One of the biggest opportunities for awkwardness is humor. Why? The foundation of what makes something humorous is compromised when one has imperfect hearing. Humor is based on the element of SURPRISE. Because the topic and content of a conversation is part of the dynamics that enable us to comprehend speech, the surprise twists and turns in humor are often lost on us with imperfect hearing, sadly.

Another challenge with humor is that so many stand-up comics talk very fast. I appreciate the closed-captioning of the comedy specials, but more often than not the words fly off the screen before I even begin to read them all.

When I don't get the joke

I ditched laughing just because others were laughing a few years ago. Inevitably, someone would turn to me and ask, "What did s/he say?" How embarrassing to tell them I had no idea. But how enlightening it was to realize how many people with "normal" hearing don't hear either!

Keep In Mind

This is something to be aware of and, when possible, compensate for when humor comes into play. If in the presence of someone hearing impaired, here are a three things you can do to ease their discomfort as far as humor is concerned.

1. If someone cracks a joke, you didn't hear it, but your hearing-impaired friend is laughing, PLEASE, PLEASE do not turn around and ask them what was said. Many of us fake laughing just to fit in. To ask us what was said is asking us to confess we didn't hear and are faking it. Really, really uncomfortable. Ask someone else if you didn't get the joke.

2. If someone cracks a joke and your hearing impaired family/friend is NOT laughing, don't make a big deal about it.

What I have found is that if someone insists I hear, the flow of the dialog comes to a screeching halt while it is explained to me. I just abhor that. All that attention focused on me, waiting for me to "get it" and laugh. Even if funny, I usually find it hard to laugh because I am uncomfortable with the fact the party has been interrupted because of me.

3. Check in with your hearing loss friend or family member about how they would like to handle any social situation or TV show BEFORE it occurs. Do they want you to make sure they hear everything? Or would they rather stay incognito? For me, I choose the latter every time. If I really want to know what was funny, I'll ask. Otherwise I'd rather be left alone.

I know this is very uncomfortable for my husband, who loves me and really wants me to participate fully in everything. That is why he wrestled for three hours with Best Buy sales people to uncover the mystery of the Netflix® closed-captioning to work on a Blu-ray player. He has learned to not insist on me hearing except on rare occasions when it is just TOO good to miss and he knows it is something I would really, really, really enjoy. In those situations, he is right, and I am grateful he made that effort for me to "get it."

So, if you have a hearing loss and don't realize why it is you do not get the jokes it is probably because of the element of surprise robbing you of the topic/content of the conversation so important for comprehension. If you are with a family member/friend with imperfect hearing, be aware of these challenges and adjust accordingly.

The Cell Phone

I don't like using the phone because it is too much work. For it to be efficient, I would have to use assistive devices. Those assistive devices require batteries, charging, etc. to keep them working. My Oticon hearing aids are compatible with a Streamer. The Streamer turns my hearing aids into a wireless head set for TV, computer and phone. That Streamer requires recharging (MORE wires to manage), hangs around my neck, and requires that I wear my hearing aids ALL the time. I don't wear my hearing aids ALL the time because when I do, I get earaches. If I push it, I will get an outer ear infection.

Not fun.

Those who know me know I prefer email or text instead of a phone call. I rarely answer my phone unless I can see who is calling and I know it is someone I can understand on the phone. Otherwise, it is a real crapshoot. Does the person calling know I have a hearing loss? If they do know, do they know how to talk to me on the phone? Do they have a good phone? Are they in a location where the transmission signal is clear? Is there background noise where they are calling from?

My voice mail used to instruct callers: "You are leaving a message for a hearing impaired person, please speak slowly, and especially enunciate numbers". What happened so often is that a person would take five excruciating slow minutes to enunciate every single word of their message that would normally only take 30 seconds, and then rattle off the phone number at the end at lightning speed! Argh! I have created an animated cartoon titled "Voice Mail" about this frequent occurrence.

Now I use Google® Voice. It is a free technology discussed in more detail in the chapter on Assistive Technology and Devices.[16]

Swimming with the Dolphins

In April 2014, I visited Cancun, Mexico during a retreat. This is what happened:

I was not expecting a huge pool with three dolphins swimming in it at this excursion. I had this romantic notion of a beautiful hidden cove in the ocean where a school of dolphins would come play with us. No way! The dolphin play was carefully orchestrated to protect us, the dolphins, and the pocket book of the vendor: Money for the many photographs. Despite the controlled conditions, it was an incredibly rewarding experience. I was enchanted with the silky flesh of our dolphin, its strength, and its intelligence.

There were about ten of us, each instructed how to do several different

---

[16] See Chapter: Additional Assistive Devices and Technology

things with the dolphin. Six are pictured here. Each image is numbered. I will explain what was going on "behind the scenes of hearing loss" in each photo. The instructor had a VERY strong accent — kiss of death for one who is hard of hearing — so I had to rely primarily on watching what the others did. Remember, no hearing aids in the water!

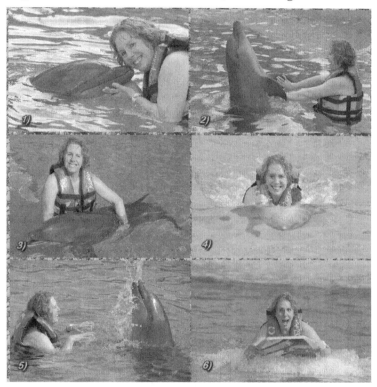

1) Mutual dolphin kiss

This provided the least amount of stress because I simply watched what everyone else did. HOWEVER, what I did not understand, and was not visible, was how to hold your hands underwater to have the dolphin's head high enough for a good smack on the "lips." I never did get a good smack on the lips. There is no good photo of that. The second part of that maneuver, the dolphin kissing ME on my cheek, pictured as #1 above, went a little better.

2) Flapping the fins

In photo #2, you see me happily flapping the dolphin's fins. The problem was the instructor and photographer kept telling me to turn my head and smile at the camera. Never happened, so I don't have a good photo of that. I eventually turned my head to the instructor figuring it was time to stop, but even then she probably said look at the camera and I just didn't understand her.

3) Hold the dolphin

I have MANY variations of photo #3 because I just couldn't get this right. Why? I could not clearly hear the instructions. Finally, they SHOWED me by physically moving my body and arms to hold the dolphin correctly.

4) Ride on dolphin's belly

I think I was most concerned with this maneuver. It required swimming way far out into the pool so there would be enough distance for a decent ride. In THIS case, I did speak up about my limitations, telling the instructor she was going to have to give me hand gestures on what to do, as I would never hear her. What they did was send out one of the workers to be besides me to make sure I climbed onto the dolphin's belly and hold the fins correctly. WHAT A RIDE I might add!

5) Dance with the dolphin

This was easy. I simply splashed my hands in the water and the dolphin emerged, spitting water and "dancing." What I did not realize is the dolphin made a noise, which I never heard.

6) Boogie board pushed by the dolphin

In this maneuver I did understand the instructions — get out there, climb on board, and hold legs/feet straight out. Easy. The bulk of the nervousness came from my concern I would not be holding my legs correctly. However, I did and was I surprised at the power and strength of the dolphin as it pushed on my foot! Absolutely exhilarating. You can see that on my face

You may be wondering, where were my friends? Did I do this excursion alone? Why didn't they help? Well, I did have a friend there who commonly helps me "hear" in challenged situations. However, I found out she was too preoccupied with her own concerns of not following the instructions correctly, and she heard perfectly well. So she forgot to help me. I didn't ask for help either.

Would I do it again? Absolutely. My recommendation, which I DID not do, would be to tell the instructors RIGHT UP FRONT that I was hearing impaired. It wasn't until I had to swim far away from the group that I finally spoke up. It is amazing that even as recent as March 2014, I STILL have a challenge fully disclosing my hearing loss when it matters.

Elevators

Elevators can make social situations and business situations potentially awkward. Nothing huge. Just slightly annoying. Here are three ways elevators have been a problem for me:

Hearing Aids Feedback

Despite the fact my aids are digital and they are not supposed to feedback (whistle/squeal), in a small tight elevator they do tend to do that. No problem if I am alone. But if with strangers, their eyes get wide and they ask, "What's that sound…?" So they don't freak and think it is a malfunction with the elevator, I usually explain it is my hearing aids that like to squeal like a pair of piglets –to make them feel less uncomfortable about my disclosure.

Elevator bells

This is not a problem if I am standing in front of a single elevator. But in a hallway with a bank of elevators, I usually do not hear an elevator bell and may miss the arrival/departure of an elevator. I have to keep a keen eye out for the LIGHT that indicates an elevator is arriving. I face this whenever I go to Kaiser for medical appointments.

Double sided elevators

This is a good topic for another cartoon. These are elevators where you enter one door to go up or down, but *exit* through elevator doors on the opposite side. I cannot begin to tell you how many times I have gone in to such elevators, and STOOD there when the elevator stopped, wondering why the door isn't opening, when all the while the door has opened and closed behind me and I didn't even know it. If someone is riding with me, they alert me. But if I'm alone, I go for an extended elevator ride.

Word Games at Parties

Games that are based on oral wordplay can be difficult for one with a hearing loss. Pictionary and Jeopardy are the two such games that caused me great distress.

Pictionary®:

In the game of Pictionary, the challenge as the person drawing an image so players can try to guess your word is that the many of the guesses being shouted at you are not audible words, they are chunks of sound! So it is hard to guide the players because you don't know what they said. Asking, "What? What?" eats away at the limited time a team has to guess the word. Not realizing this problem ahead of time, I placed myself in a very embarrassing and uncomfortable position at a party playing Pictionary. This is captured in the cartoon I created called "Pictionary"

Jeopardy®:

The Jeopardy game is not a problem to watch on TV or to answer as a "contestant"; the problem is being the Alex Trebek – that is – listening for the right answer (or should I say "question", as is the case in Jeopardy). Several years ago, while still working at UCLA, I put together a Jeopardy game for a holiday party. All the questions and answers had to do with our jobs — research administration. So there I sat in the middle of 40 or more people facilitating this Jeopardy game; being the Alex Trebek. Instead of individuals playing against one another, teams were playing against one another — but only one person could speak on behalf of their team. Well, it was a disaster. Individuals would give their answer and I would have to ask questions to clarify what they said — which, a few times, GAVE the answer away. It was so humiliating! I turned to a colleague about half way through and said, "You know, I shouldn't be doing this."
She replied, "Yea, I know." But she didn't offer to take over. I suffered through the best I could — trying to ignore the occasional grumble or "boo" when a team got an unfair advantage due to my "clarification"

process. When the game was over, I went into my office shut the door and cried.

If you or someone you know, has a hearing loss and are invited to participate in an oral word-play game, proceed with caution. I would not go into such a game without forewarning the players that I'll likely not be able to play due to my hearing loss. But in most cases I don't even do that. I just decline the opportunity to play. Or suggest Scrabble® as an alternative.

Misunderstanding Similar Sounding Words

In my cartoons called the "Hearing Impaired Chorus Girl" and "New Hearing Aids" a young woman is unaware she is misunderstanding and mispronouncing words. For example, in one cartoon she is in an elevator and shares with a colleague she just got new a new hearing aid. "What kind is it?" her colleague asks. Looking down at her watch, she responds "9:00 am." The chorus girl is an extremely exaggerated truism of misunderstanding the words in songs.

These hearing mishaps put others in an awkward position. Do they tell her or not? If they do, she may likely feel awkward, or become defensive. It can be a no win situation.

Getting the Address Wrong

I have had some serious challenges when it comes to addresses! Friends and family give me an address over the phone and I THINK I got it right. In fact, I would SWEAR I got it right. But, there I'd be wandering all over Southern California looking for an address that doesn't exist, or winding up somewhere other than where I'm supposed to be. Even if I read the address back to someone, if he/she were not listening carefully they would absently say, "Yea, that's right" even though I just read them the wrong address or street name.

I captured this in yet another cartoon titled "The Address"

The numbers "1" and "9" and "2" and "3" are most problematic for me. Remember, I am only hearing a piece of sound. As for street names, since there are many sounds I do not hear fully hear it isn't hard to see how I can get the name of a street wrong. Suppose the street name is Barton Avenue. All I hear of that is a piece of the "a" the "r" and the "n". It could be any variations of those sounds. If I think I heard "Carson Avenue", well, guess who is not going to arrive on time – or at all.

Workarounds

If hearing impaired or interacting with someone with a hearing loss, it is best to put that address in writing — and verify it. This is pretty easy these days thanks to technology.

Email: I will often ask people to email the address of where I am supposed to be. There is no "hearing" to deal with then. Of course, I have to hope the sender does not put a typo in the address.

GPS Navigation Systems: I so appreciate the navigation systems available in cars and on cell phones. If I do hear an address incorrectly or someone sends me an address with a typo, putting it into a GPS system (or even one of the Internet maps like Google® Maps, MapQuest, etc). helps to clarify if that address does not look correct and enables me to be proactive against getting lost.

As an aside, the voice feature of a GPS navigation system is not good for me by itself — I must see the guidance as well. I'm amazed how "right" and "left" sound almost the same to me when dictated by the electronic voice of a GPS. Of course, if I make a wrong turn I can hear "When possible, please make a legal U turn." I prefer to get it right the first time!

Cell phones – especially Smartphones: I think Smartphones are the best invention since computers. They serve us all so well in a myriad of ways — especially if we are hearing, impaired. Here are ways the cell phone can assist in getting addresses right:

Email: (that contains the address) can be accessed from a cell phone. If the email has the full address and you are viewing it via a Smartphone, that address is often hyperlinked. Click on the address and presto, a map pops up.

Text messaging: Ask the person to text the address. This is especially handy when you realize you DO have the wrong address and quickly need the right one. Provided you can get a hold of someone, that someone can text you the right address immediately.

We can SWEAR we heard something right...but we didn't. With the use of email, GPS systems and cell phones, we can verify those addresses before hitting the road.

Asking "What?"

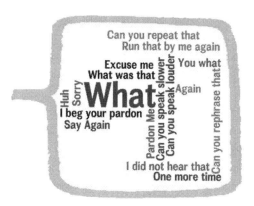

In the book I mentioned previously, *Shouting Won't Help: Why I–and 50 Million Other Americans–Can't Hear You,* author Katherine Bouton shares how her husband asked her to find alternatives to the question "What?" when she needed him to repeat something — which was most everything. "What" began to feel a bit like Chinese water torture after a while.

With strangers, asking "what" every time they say something can be misconstrued as questioning their opinion. Trust me. It happens. Not often. Nevertheless, it happens. If a person is not secure about himself or what he is saying, your "What?" can induce some pretty strong reactions.

All in all, it's a good idea to have some alternatives up your sleeve. I have come up with several alternatives to the flat, "What?" Here they are:

Alternatives to Asking "What?"

- Huh?

- Say again?
- Pardon me?
- What was that?
- I didn't hear that.
- I didn't catch that
- Can you repeat that?
- Can you rephrase that?
- Can you speak slower?
- Can you speak louder?
- One more time, please.
- Say what?
- You what?
- I'm sorry?
- Say again?
- I beg your pardon?
- Run that by me again?
- Excuse me?

The one I most often use is "Pardon me?" It just sounds, well, more sophisticated than "What?" or "Huh?" Of course, with people who really know me, I don't say anything. My face tells them I didn't understand and they repeat themselves without my having to ask. If they repeat themselves a couple of times and I still don't get it, then I may ask them to rephrase it. When all else fails, I may ask them to write it down.

It all depends on the situation, the person, and how I am feeling.

Misperceptions of Who I Am

If I don't hear at all, or don't hear correctly, my "wrong" response can be misinterpreted as not caring or being aloof or worse. This can be a real problem in the workplace. This is what happened to me at my first job, before I started wearing hearing aids regularly.

An elderly Black man thought I was a racist because I didn't answer him when he spoke to me as I passed him in the hall. He began to cop a real attitude with me, which I assumed was because of my disability. We had a good laugh and became good friends once we discovered the truth.

Confusion

Did you get the Pies?

I still am not sure exactly what was said in response to my question, "Did you get the pies?" but there were ultimately four discussions about who was going to get what pies and when to take to a dinner party my sister-in-law was organizing. It was October and we were visiting my in-laws in Vermont. It is tradition that we contribute pies from Mazza's, a delightful farm store, bakery and greenhouse just a very short walk from my father-in-law's home. I believe the confusion began when my father-in-law (who has a tendency to speak as if his teeth were clenched) answered that he had picked up a pumpkin pie already and would pick up the second pie in the morning. I, with my hearing loss and hearing in chunks, surmised that the both pies had been purchased already. During a second discussion, I guess it was clarified that the second pie had NOT yet been purchased — and I, once again, not fully hearing the discussion due to my hearing loss, surmised that no pies had been purchased. So, the next morning when I went to get coffee at Mazza's, I had the baker set aside two pies to pick up later. One pumpkin. One apple. Well, there was quite a bit of confusion and MORE discussion at the store when my father-in-law went to purchase that second pie and he learned that two pies were on hold already. I apologized to everyone — the confusion was caused by my not making sure I understood the entire discussion initially.

The end of the story is we did finally have one pumpkin pie and one apple pie to take to the party. After a while this was so comical it became an on-going family joke. But the joke was on me....

These are just awkward moments. Here are some disastrous, or near disastrous moments that I and others with a hearing loss, have experienced.

Disastrous Moments

Spilling Secrets or Surprises

This just happened recently. (I have changed the location and situation to protect the innocent). I was visiting a friend in her office. My business partner, Circe, was with me too. One of my friend's associates popped in, said something excitedly to her, and walked out. My friend looked at me and explained, "We are going to a party." I heard that. Then she said something that I didn't hear and I started to bluff until I paid closer attention to her body language and facial expressions and the body language and facial expressions of Circe's response. Whatever I did not hear was important. I spoke up, "I'm sorry. I didn't hear the last thing you said." My friend responded, "It is a *surprise* party for someone in the receptionist area, so don't say anything on the way out."

Ok. You get the picture here. If I had not clarified that this was a secret, I could have easily said, "Have fun at the party" on my way out. Not good!

Losing a Bid

I read about a man who refused to get hearing aids until one fateful day at the office. He was sitting at a table with competitors bidding on a job. It was a big and important construction job. He did not hear the correct amount of a bid of his competitor and came in with an unreasonably higher bid. Result? His company lost the job and his boss lost his patience. He made the hearing-impaired elderly employee retire, as the company could not afford any future hearing mishaps. The resistant employee finally agreed to hearing aids after that.

Insensitive Response

In another book, I read about a hearing-impaired woman who was having lunch with her friend. Her friend told her that her husband had been diagnosed with cancer. She did not hear what was said, bluffed and responded with a smile and "That's nice" and changed the subject. Her friend got up and walked out.

Gross Misinterpretation

Many years ago, I was at a party. I had brought my beautiful girlfriend, Kathy, single and needing some social activity. I knew most everyone at this party, so was quite comfortable. Also attending the party was a couple, not married, but living together — Cindy and Joe. Joe was busy chatting away. I wasn't getting much of what he was saying, but I SWORE I heard him say something about marrying Cindy. Later Cindy pulled me into a bedroom and with great emphasis and energy said a bunch of words in a short of whisper shout that I could not hear. On with the bluff, I ASSUMED she was excited about Joe's remark about marrying her. So I sat there nodding my head in agreement with what she was saying.

The next morning I received a phone call from Cindy. She was angry, crying and quite upset. I was shocked, "What's wrong?" I inquired. "I'm upset about all that flirting that was going on between your friend Kathy and my Joe. You agreed with me that it was pretty obvious….." Ooops! I stammered as I explained to Cindy that I bluffed hearing Joe talking and THOUGHT he said something about marrying her; and worst, I bluffed hearing her assuming she was excited at what I thought Joe said. I was pretty embarrassed. And sorry. I caused great distress for Cindy. Cindy lambasted Joe about his flirtatious nature. My friend Kathy was not welcome to another party where Cindy and Joe may be present. Disaster.

Distracted

One of my favorite characters in the early days of Saturday Night Live was Roseanne Roseannadanna, played by Gilda Radner. She did a spiel once about an elegant woman walking out of the bathroom with toilet paper dragging behind her that had been caught on her high heel.

"Boy!" I thought to myself, "that would be awful. I sure hope that never happens to me."

Well the WORST did happen to me — 3 times

All three times, it happened when I was not focused — distracted and looking "forward" rather than being in the now. I do not hear paper rustle, even with aids, especially toilet seat covers. THREE times in a rush, I accidently got the toilet seat cover caught in my pants and walked out into public with it waving behind me. Fortunately, in two of those incidents not many people saw it. At work, someone pointed it out to me the moment I walked out of the stall. In another incident, the seat cover became visible when I took my coat off while getting into the car and a nice couple came over and told me about it. What is SO disturbing about THAT was that I had just given a 45-minute talk at their church. Thank GOD, the visit to the restroom was AFTER I finished the talk, and that my coat covered me so no one saw it as I exited the premises. But, there was one time when I wasn't so lucky. I was at a casino in Las Vegas. I went to the restroom and it must have been an HOUR before someone came up to me and told me I had a toilet seat cover hanging off my butt. I wanted to shoot myself. Today I squat, or I stay super focused to make sure EVERYTHING is getting flushed down that toilet.

Oblivious

In the 1980's, I volunteered as a helper for a sweet man who was running for a position on the Los Angeles City Council. Come the election night I am running around all smiley, happy, totally oblivious to the fact that he had LOST the election. I could not understand the conversation of those around me. I presume someone must have told me. I bluffed hearing and made a complete ASS of myself. Now I understand why a car full of them looked at me as if I was from another planet when the event was over.

In conclusion:

All in the day and life of having a hearing loss. Some days it really upsets me. Other days, I take it in stride. What's my preference? That none of this happen. I wish I did not have a hearing loss!

Chapter 12 References and Resources:

Bouton, K. (2013). *Shouting Won't Help - Why I - and 50 Million Other Americans - Can't Hear You.* New York: Sarah Crichton Books.

Photography for Dolphin Excursion:

http://www.dolphindiscovery.com/playa-del-carmen/dolphin-encounter.asp

Cartoon: "Voice Mail" - https://www.youtube.com/edit?o=U&video_id=5KuotzeMEAA

Cartoon: Pictionary: https://www.youtube.com/watch?v=4rrtnEsH1_4

Cartoon: "Hearing Impaired Chorus Girl" - https://www.youtube.com/watch?v=CEAy13vkk9A

Cartoon: "New Hearing Aids" - https://www.youtube.com/watch?v=pnSooQhW8Zg

Cartoon: "The Address" - https://www.youtube.com/watch?v=jR-ZihRtgqo

Linnaea Mallette

CHAPTER 13:
HEARING LOSS MYTHS

"Don't whisper. Also, don't shout. And if you... speak... like... this... I will punch you."
– Kelly Dougher

The three myths about hearing loss that I find most prevalent have to do with

1. Hearing aids;
2. Lip Reading
3. Shouting

Let's examine these more closely:

Hearing Aids

Myth: If they are wearing hearing aids, they can hear. Wrong!

Hearing aids help, but they do not restore one to perfect hearing.

Most of the people I know who have to wear hearing aids do not have "normal" hearing as a result of wearing them. I sure don't. In fact, at times they interfere with what hearing I do have — like in noisy situations.

In the chapter about hearing aids,[17] we met Alex, who, in his 50's was fitted for hearing aids. He was crushed when he realized that the hearing aids helped, but far from restored his perfect hearing. Well, that story continues here…

Alex's family and friends, seeing he had hearing aids, fully expected that he could now hear normally. They ceased making the extra effort to ensure communication (being close, looking at him, speaking slightly louder and enunciating words). Well, they, along with Alex, were deeply disappointed and frustrated when they discovered that Alex still had a difficult time hearing. Sure, the aids helped, but they did not restore him to normal hearing.

---

[17] See Chapter: Hearing Aids – Saving Grace –Necessary Evil

Of course, family and friends aren't the only ones surprised by this myth. Most people assume that if a person has a hearing aid on s/he is going to hear okay. And more often than not, the extra effort to communicate is ditched because, after all, "s/he is wearing hearing-aids." This is not an assumption you want your employees to practice with important customers or clients.

When I conduct talks and trainings to those who serve the community, I am emphatic about this: assume that when people are wearing hearing aids THEY ARE still hearing impaired. The larger the aids, in fact, the more attention one must pay to the conversation. I suggest applying my "CPR" to save the conversation from dying and the relationship strained or ruined[18].

Lip Reading

Myth: If they can read lips, they can comprehend what we are saying. Wrong.

Lip reading helps, but in and of itself, it is not enough for complete communication.

Lip reading as defined by Wikipedia: "… is a technique of understanding speech by visually interpreting the movements of the lips, face and tongue when normal sound is not available."

You have seen it many times in James Bond type of movies. The spy is sitting in a noisy bar and reading the lips of their adversary sitting on the other side of the room. And they are getting every single word.

Ha! That's Hollywood! Full of myths and fantasies.

Studies show that the MOST skilled of lip readers can only comprehend a mere 30%-40% of a conversation relying solely on the lips. Facial expressions, body language, the topic of a conversation or circumstances, and how well you know the person you are speaking to, all add to the ability to comprehend what a person is saying when reading lips.

The challenge in lip reading is that many sounds look the same on lips.

---

[18] See Chapter: CPR for Hearing Loss

For example, P, B and G, all look alike on lips.

To fully appreciate how words can look the same on lips (and for a good laugh) visit http://badlipreading.com.

But, like hearing aids — lip reading certainly HELPS. I get frustrated if my lip reading is thwarted by things like:

Long bushy mustaches

Hands in front of the mouth

Mouths full of food

Dark environments

Super exaggerated lip movements (doesn't help)

Person not looking at me

Back light causing the person to be silhouetted

Group discussions (not knowing where to look when someone starts to talk)

Lose dentures that flap while a person is talking (that is like lip reading in double vision).

Group discussions are a challenge in a classroom setting — especially as a trainer. A person speaks up to ask a question or make a comment, but I don't know where the voice is coming from. I always ask people to raise their hand as they are speaking so I know where to LOOK to then take advantage of reading them — not only their lips — but their face and body too.

When communicating with someone with a hearing loss, if you see them reading your lips, know that your lips are just part of the total cues they are taking in to facilitate their successful communication with you. When you recognize someone is reading your lips, slow down just a bit, and enunciate just a tad more. Exaggerated lips don't help. Just a slight emphasis is helpful.

Shouting

Myth: If I shout, they will hear me.

Wrong

Shouting is not necessary and does not help. Slightly louder, slower, and a bit more articulation does help.

My favorite analogy for shouting is to go home, turn on your TV to a foreign channel, and turn off the captioning. There. Now. You hear, but you don't understand. Right? If you turn the TV up real loud will you now understand what they are saying? No. The words are still incomprehensible.

That is what it is like for us with higher degrees of hearing loss. Shouting simply does not help.

What does help is talking as clearly and distinctly as possible, facing the person, so the dynamics of hearing[19] can be fully utilized.

So given this information, what do you do if interacting with, or as a person with a hearing loss? While there are many tips, the next chapter covers what I consider the most important ones. I call them "CPR" because they can save a conversation from dying on the vine.

In conclusion:

Practicing any of these three myths will likely negatively affect communication with a hearing-impaired person.

Chapter 13 References and Resources:

Wikipedia. (n.d).. *Lip Reading*. Retrieved from Wikipedia:
    http://en.wikipedia.org/wiki/Lip_reading

Hopkins, J. (n.d).. *Deaf/Hard of Hearing*. Retrieved from Office of Student Diability Services:
http://web.jhu.edu/disabilities/faculty/types_of_disabilities/deafness.html

Mehrabian, P. A. (n.d).. *Mehrabian's communication research*. Retrieved October 21, 2014, from kaaj.com: http://www.kaaj.com/psych/smorder.html

---

[19] See Chapter: Dynamics of Hearing

CHAPTER 14:
DYNAMICS OF HEARING

"What you do speaks so loudly that I cannot hear what you say." – Emerson

A comment I often hear when I am successfully participating in a conversation is, "I thought you were deaf. How did you hear that?" I explain I am not totally deaf, and I rely much on the dynamics of hearing. Dynamics we all use in comprehending speech. These dynamics are capitalized on, of course, by those of us with hearing loss. They are:

- Topic of a conversation
- Body language and facial expressions
- Voice and tonality

Topic and Content of a Conversation

Have you ever been in a conversation with someone when suddenly, mid-stream, out of the blue, for no reason at all, they shift gears and talk about something else totally unrelated to the current discussion? What is your first response? "Huh?" "What?" "What ARE you talking about?" Is that because you have a hearing loss? No. It is because much of what you were previously hearing was based on the topic and content of the conversation. When the conversation topic shifted without any warning, the subsequent verbiage didn't "match", what the brain had been expecting and interpreting. For a brief time, you are at a loss until you know the topic and content of the new conversation. This often happens so fast you may not even be aware you are doing it. But we all do it.

Here is an exaggerated example for the sake of illustration:

Imagine you are standing in line at a convenience store and someone from a foreign land with an extremely strong accent comes up behind you and starts a conversation. The accent is so strong you strain hard; eyes squinted, in an effort to understand what this nice person is enthusiastically saying. Suddenly you hear something that sounds like, "Magic Kingdom." With THAT piece of information, you listen some more and, indeed, that is what the person is talking about — his recent visit to Disneyland. Armed with the topic, you are able to comprehend the words much better; a whole lot more. Your brain is chock full of information about Disneyland that fills in the blanks, so to speak, of what you may not clearly understand from this foreign visitor. By-and-large, with the topic and content known, you have enough to participate in the conversation.

Now, suppose this foreign visitor is chatting on a topic of which you know NOTHING — like nuclear physics. With no data bank of knowledge in your brain to draw upon to help fill in the gaps of what you do not comprehend, you probably are going to explain politely to the enthusiastic visitor that you are not able to understand him and end the conversation. Or bluff…

Topic and content of a conversation. It was the ONLY way I was able to host my own radio show for 18 months a few years ago.

The broadcast was conducted from my home with a good mic that had a jack for a headset and Skype®[20] The company I went with was a high-end provider, TogiNet. I had a live person monitoring everything on the other end while the show was going on. I had a control panel where the TogiNet employee and I could type messages back and forth to one another during the show. I was very careful about who I picked to be on my show. Many I already knew personally or professionally. I would have the guests send me details about their topics so I had that benefit of the "topic and content" dynamics working for me. There were not many people on my show with a speech impediment or strong accent. There were a few, and the fact I could not understand them is evident in the show. Even with the best connection, guest and conversation, when I listen to previous recordings there are several incidences when I did not hear correctly and the guest gracefully worked around it.

How can this knowledge serve those of us who have a hearing loss or are interacting with someone with a hearing loss? Make sure the TOPIC, and the CONTENT, of a conversation is clear. After 2-3 tries if the other person is not following along, write it down or create a draft text message on your Smartphone and show it to the person. You

---

[20] See Chapter: Additional Assistive Devices and Technology

will see the light go on in the eyes and relief spread over the face. S/he can now participate in the conversation, even if minimally.

A wonderful audiologist whose husband is hearing impaired told me that when they are out to dinner with friends, she always clues him in when the topic of a conversation has shifted so he has a better opportunity to stay connected with the party. She will turn to him and say, "Honey, we are now talking about the movie 'Terminator.'" He smiles, nods, and the conversation continues — with him.

Take away here? When conversing with someone, whether they have perfect hearing or not, make sure the topic and content of the conversation is clear right from the get-go. If you are discussing a topic for which the listener(s) are not familiar, be prepared to slow down and repeat yourself. Not because they have hearing loss, but because they are not familiar with the topic or content of THAT conversation. The brain needs time to assimilate information. This is true for those with or without a hearing loss.

Body Language and Facial Expressions

As a professional speaker, I know how important it is to make sure my body language and facial expressions match what I am saying. I spend considerable time on that topic on my site about public speaking. As a person with a hearing loss, the language of the body and face is essential to my ability to comprehend what a person is saying to me. Prior to the days of closed captioning on TV, much of what I gleaned from the shows was based on body language and facial expressions, and I did pretty darn good!

In a book titled, *Nonverbal Communication*, Dr. Albert Mehrabian, Professor Emeritus of Psychology at UCLA, claims facial expressions are almost eight times as powerful as the words used. He explains that words only count for 7% of our message. He further explains that 55% of our message is conveyed by our body language. Look at these two sets of images. You can get a pretty good idea of what the face and body depicts without a single word spoken:

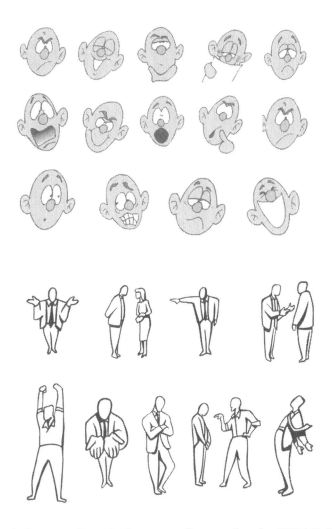

These statistics, may I remind you, are for people who HEAR. We do this unconsciously. But when communicating with someone with imperfect hearing, be conscious and make sure that the person is looking at you before you speak so s/he has the benefit of "reading" you. All of you.

The Lips

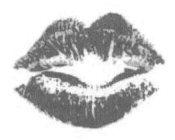

Lip reading (also known as speech reading) merits its own entry. I go into detail about the myths associated with lip reading in another chapter[21] But for this chapter, it is important to note that the lips are a part of reading the face. While only the best lip readers can get 40% of a conversation if reading lips alone, they, in combination with body, face and eyes, help to connect the dots and get a conversation — or at least the essence of it.

Voice and Tonality

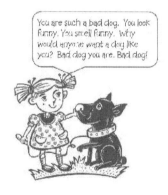

When I was younger and I had dogs, I always got a big kick out of saying awful things to them in a sweet voice and watching them respond positively. They were responding not to my words but to the tone of my voice. That is why in addition to body language and facial expressions, the voice and tonality conveys so much more than words.

---

[21] See Chapter: Hearing Loss Myths"

Dr. Albert Mehrabian reported that 38% of a message is relayed by our voice. Have you not noticed how one's voice can reveal what a person is feeling deep down inside? Note how your voice conveys enthusiasm or boredom; pleasure or pain; sincerity or sarcasm; and happiness or sadness. The sound of your voice can be used to help a person with a hearing loss understand what you are saying. You might even exaggerate the tone of your voice a bit to facilitate comprehension of your words.

Capitalize on the dynamics of topic and content — communication will be more easily received and achieved — no matter whom you are chatting with.

In conclusion:

Only 7% of communication is achieved through exchange of words. While a small percentage, we do need to know what those words are about! The other 93% is body language, facial expressions, voice and tonality. Capitalize on this as a person with a hearing loss or when communicating with a person with a hearing loss by:

1. Being 3–5 feet away from the person, with whom you are having a conversation.
2. Looking at one another before the conversation begins.
3. Making sure the topic of the conversation is clear from the get-go.
4. Accentuating, not over dramatizing, body language and voice during the conversation.

Chapter 14 References and Resources:

Podcasts of Linnaea's Read My Lips Tips for Success Radio Show archived at **http://www.LinnaeaMallette.com**

Chapman, A. (2004). *Mehrabian's Communication Research*. Retrieved 2013, from Business Balls:
http://www.businessballs.com/mehrabiancommunications.htm

Linnaea's site about public speaking: http://www.Kiss-Speaking-Tips.com

CHAPTER 15:
CONVERSING WITH HEARING IMPAIRED INDIVIDUALS

"The single biggest problem in communication is the illusion that it has taken place." – George Bernard Shaw

These are tips and techniques you can use when interacting with a person with a hearing loss, or explaining to others if you are the person with the hearing loss.

CPR

We already know that shouting does not help when talking with someone with a hearing loss. Especially if you are shouting right into their ear and they do not have the benefit of reading your body language, facial expressions, eyes and lips.

I have come up with a simple technique you can use when you recognize you are communicating with a person with a hearing loss. Encapsulated in the simple acronym "CPR" for ease in memory and recall — and the fact that it can rescue a conversation from dying.

"CPR" stands for:

C: Close

Have the person close to you and looking at you. 3-5 feet is best. This enables the person with the loss to capitalize on the dynamics of hearing[22], that is, read your body language, facial expressions (which includes the lips)and hear more readily the tone of your voice — which accounts for 94% of hearing — even for those with perfect hearing!

P: Pause

Those of us who do public speaking are taught the importance of the pause. There is a slight delay while the brain receives sound and tries to

---

[22] See Chapter: Dynamics of Hearing

make sense of it — more so with those of us with a hearing loss. The pause between sentences enables the listeners to ABSORB the message we have just given them. This is doubly critical when communicating with a person with diminished hearing. If you can communicate using shorter sentences with pauses in-between, communication is easier. Here is an example:

You might say:

"I am going to the store to pick up some milk. I am making ice cream tonight for dessert."

If you said that fast with no pauses, I probably would not get it on first pass. Especially if it is not connected to a topic, we have already been discussing.

"What?" I'd ask.

Applying the pause would sound like this:

"I am going to the store. [pause] I am picking up some milk. [pause] I am making ice cream tonight for dessert."

Ah, at this juncture, my eyes would probably light up and I'd say, "Oh cool! Can I join you?"

If you do this aloud, you can feel how much easier this is to hear and comprehend. Less work to hear for anyone!

R: Repeat and Rephrase

I created a cartoon titled "Soup or Salad" based on the real experience of a person with a hearing loss at a restaurant. The waiter kept repeating the question, "Would you like soup or salad?" and the customer kept answering "yes" because what she heard the waiter ask is, "Would you like a *super salad*?" I think all those in the service industry should receive training on communicating with customers who have trouble hearing! Especially when hearing is further compromised in the noisy environment of a restaurant! When a person says "what" or clearly did not hear you correctly, repeat. After two attempts, try rephrasing. This is how that looks:

You might say:

"I am going to the store"

"What?" says me.

You apply "R" and repeat.

"I am going to the store."

"Pardon me?" is still my response accompanied with a slightly twisted face.

You then apply the "R" but this time REPHRASE:

"I am going to the market."

"OHHHHH," I say as I finally get it.

Communication achieved!

The waiter depicted in the cartoon could have rephrased his question after two failed attempts and ask, "Would you prefer a bowl of soup or a salad?" No confusion there!

So when communication is compromised, for whatever reason, try the CPR technique to rescue it from dying; leaving you and the listener frustrated.

In conclusion:

Communication with, or as, a person with a hearing loss takes caring, attention and work — for both sides.

Chapter 15 References and Resources:

Cartoon, "Soup or Salad" – YouTube;

https://www.youtube.com/watch?v=WxMQE60VkeM

CHAPTER 16:
PERSPECTIVE OF FRIENDS

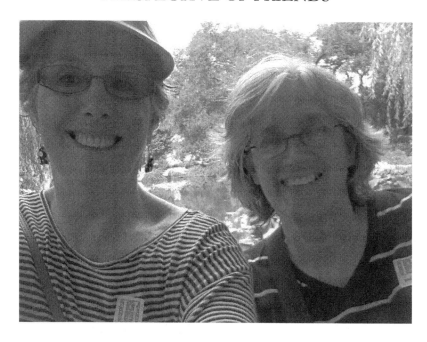

My business partner and dear friend Circe Denyer (pictured above) wrote three posts about her interactions with me as a friend with a hearing loss. They are repeated below.

Post 1: I Take Responsibility

"I learned how Linnaea can 'mis-hear' and require a repeat of the sentence to understand it. I now also understand that this is my responsibility in the conversation. I can slow down. I can enunciate and use words that contain easy to discern components. Linnaea does not hear "ch", so the words I choose using those may not be understood. In knowing that, repeating without slowing down frustrates the conversation and reduces the quality of it for her. When she does not "get" what I say, it is my fault, even though she is the one with impaired hearing.

I drive when we go places together. She gets an opportunity to talk, which I can hear while driving and she can read my lips when I respond. Again, I must remember to speak clearly, even though she is reading me for understanding.

I hardly ever focus on sounds coming at me from my environment when I am alone. I "know" I will be able to tell if there is something coming my way that I must give my attention to, such as a car in a parking lot, or an announcement over the PA. Linnaea does not have that luxury. Some sounds are indiscernible until they are right on top of her, so I make sure I am not "zoned" out while we are together."

Note: I, Linnaea, believe it is MY responsibility too when a person is interacting with me. It is my responsibility to be looking at her/him and making an effort to understand when s/he is making an effort. My husband will often not even begin to talk until I have stopped what I am doing and give him my full attention. It is also my responsibility to let strangers know I have a hearing loss.

Post 2: I Minimize Inference

For someone like Linnaea who doesn't have the benefit (or in many cases the luxury) of hearing discussions going on around her, there is a lot of 'common knowledge' that she may not be aware of because she has never heard about it. An example is when she needed cash, and she did not realize she could obtain cash by using her bankcard at a grocery store checkout. I wondered how I learned about this, and I realized it is because I HEARD people talking about and doing that at check stands for years. Linnaea does not hear ambient talking — the conversations around her that are not directly engaging her.

And how about talking on the phone?

We all have had the experience of a person on the other end of our email communication misinterpreting the spirit in which we sent the message. That is because the email contains no inference. Emoticons help convey what you really mean. When communicating with a person with imperfect hearing, inferences and subtle tones of words are missed altogether. That means our conversation can be taken the wrong way. For this reason, it is SO important to use more descriptive words and language when communicating with a person with a hearing loss — ESPECIALLY if it is via the phone. So much is conveyed by the body and face. When it comes to the phone, I have found that it is better to stick to the facts, be brief, and go slow. Short deliberate statements are best.

I save the playful stuff until the person is in my physical presence. Here is an example:

If I am going to JOKE with Linnaea, saying something like, "Oh sure, you are just a big liar…"OR "Oh sure, I believe THAT…" or something else playful, the inflection of my voice is missing — and the joke can be lost. I have learned it is best to never use a joke like that via the phone, and if in person, save that joke until she is in the same room with me, facing me, and she can see my smiling face. You may think that the phone transmits the inflection and therefore the INTENT, but cell phones are unclear, dependent on the closest microwave tower, and not good for communication where subtlety is used. It takes EFFORT for me to do this. I spend a great deal of my time communicating with people over the phone. Add to that I am a sarcastic teaser, and BINGO! I WILL BE MISUNDERSTOOD!!!

A person with any form of hearing loss does not pick up inference. Inference is used in jokes and sarcasm. I love to joke and I love to be sarcastic. I learned that much of a joke's impact and understanding comes from inference. Without it, the joke is never understood. Inference is also used in day-to-day relationships. We use tone and subtlety to connect in intimate and close relationships. If you are in a relationship with someone who is hearing impaired, use language not inference to connect and enjoy the companionship. Here is an example, using the situation mentioned above about the cash from the supermarket. When I heard Linnaea say she needed cash and the bank was too far away; if I said, "just get it from the supermarket", I would be inferring she use the ATM at checkout. Realizing she didn't know about the ATM checkout option, because unlike me, she never heard others in line doing that, I would say instead: "The Supermarket lets you get cash back at checkout, using the keypad." More words, less confusion, better communication.

Don't use jokes unless they are written. The hurtful effect of missing out on the joke is easily avoided if you understand this side of hearing loss."

Post 3: From Phone to Text

"I am a tech oriented person who LIVES on the phone and the adjustment from phone to text has been perfect in our friendship.

- I text instead of call.
- I Skype® instead of call.
- I use more words to explain what I need/want/care to express to make sure it is properly understood. Otherwise, I find myself laughing at the results of the conversation. Hearing loss can cause some interesting misinterpretations!
- I wait. This is the most important part of the conversation transmission via text or Skype. When a text is received and I do not respond immediately, the text gets 'out of order'. Thus, the conversation can mean something entirely different.

Linnaea has a favorite quote and it means much to me. George Bernard Shaw said 'The single biggest problem in communication is the illusion that it has taken place.'

When I wait for the PAUSE in the chat or text, I can figure out if there are multiple questions or parts to it.

I use this format: SUBJECT: ANSWER

An example:

Text from Linnaea: 'Did you look at the post for CatWows? I just love the way the Maude video turned out.'

'I am heading out for coffee.'

My too quick response: Yes.'

What is that response in reaction to? If I had waited...

'CatWows: Yes, Coffee: see ya later."

The latter, fuller response, is a better conversation than my hasty "yes", and is less likely to be misunderstood.

It is not just about the text/chat as opposed to phone. It is about the quality of communication and what is going to be best understood in the long term — especially when communicating with someone with a hearing loss. This makes it fun, interesting and with less 'illusion'. I take the stand that the quality of conversations is my responsibility. I hear. She cannot. I get it. She has the hearing loss.

I apologize when I forget. So many times, my friend does such a good job 'listening' and reading my lips that I get carried away and slip back into the habit of talking too fast and speaking while not facing her. I am aware that the understanding is on me, I am not the one who cannot hear."

Do I appreciate Circe's friendship? YOU BET!

In conclusion:

The best method to communicate with your hearing impaired family member, friend or co-worker is to be educated and practice what works best — for both parties.

Linnaea Mallette

CHAPTER 17:
MORE THAN MEETS THE EYE.

"There are so many people, deaf or otherwise disabled, who are so talented but overlooked or not given a chance to even get their foot in the door."
-Marlee Matlin

One out of every five Americans has a disability. I have observed as a person with a physical disability that society, on the whole, has a ways to go when accepting people with disabilities. Many tend to ignore or avoid us, as if something is WRONG with us.

Individuals with disabilities are not disabled. Just like everyone else, there are things we can do, and things we cannot do. The difference, however, is that people with disabilities tend to *focus on what they can do, not what they cannot do.* A good example is the husband of an acquaintance who was a "stud muffin" in high school — top of his game athletically, who was in an accident shortly after he graduated that left him paralyzed from the neck down. That did not stop him from graduating with honors from Harvard and Yale. He is a self-made millionaire through his keen ability to manage money, especially stocks and mutual funds.

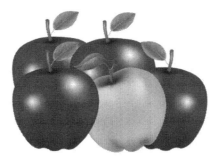

I love the analogy offered by Kathie Snow on her website titled *Disability is Natural.* She explains that one out of every five apples is green. Yet, one does not think of the green apple as a problem needing to be fixed. Green apples are naturally different. Not wrong. Just different. If we, as a society, could accept the differences of a person with a disability with the same casualness, we accept the difference of the green apple, the quality of life for the disabled would be greatly enhanced.

That is usually not the case. I think it is primarily because people are uncomfortable around us. They do not know what to do. To escape the possibility of embarrassing themselves, or us, they avoid us. Most of us with a physical disability understand that people need time to become comfortable around us. On most days, we are patient with, and appreciative of, any awkward attempts individuals may make to be helpful or connect. However, there are certainly days when we do wish, more than anything, we could be viewed and treated as "normal."

Getting Comfortable

It takes deliberate education and practice to become comfortable around a person with a disability. Even I, a person with a disability, found it excruciatingly uncomfortable to be around others with a different form of physical disability. Anyone in a wheel chair with something other than a broken leg was downright scary to me. And blind people? I SEE to hear, so I could not even get my thoughts around being able to communicate without seeing! I understand the discomfort of being around a person with a physical disability. How pleased I was when, I, while serving as a District leader for Toastmasters, visited Braille Toastmasters — a room full of blind members, and I was not only comfortable, I had a blast. I was equally pleased when I visited a Disabled American Veterans event where over half of those in attendance were men in wheelchairs with one or both legs missing and I felt perfectly at ease.

I owe this radical shift in my perception to my involvement in Toastmasters, where I got up close and personal to many individuals with disabilities. I think the most important thing I learned from being in Toastmasters is that EVERYONE has a disability of some sort, potentially disabling them temporarily — or permanently — from fully participating, fully succeeding, in some or all aspects of their life. Being too tall, too short, too smart, too dumb, too fat, to slow, too fast might be a disability. Perhaps being White, Black, Asian, having a strong accent is a disability. The child of a dysfunctional parent or a veteran who has survived the ravages of a war can be emotionally disabled for life. The unexpected, untimely death of a loved one, a broken heart, diagnosis of a deadly disease, all are disabilities of a sort. Disability can be real or imagined, but it affects the way one responds to others, the way they see themselves in the world.

Hero's Heart

My 25 plus years listening to hundreds of stories from speakers from all walks of life has convinced me that we are all much more alike than different. We all are on a hero's journey, with a hero's heart, wanting to contribute, to be of value, to be loved, to be respected, to be accepted, to belong. I recall the most moving scene in the movie, A Beautiful Mind, is when all those professors were giving John Forbes (played by Russell Crowe) their pens, signifying their respect and acceptance of him.

Helen Keller, blind and deaf at birth, said, "The highest result of education is tolerance." I say it is even more. Education about the variety of disabilities and working to become comfortable around individuals with them adds a depth to your character that would be impossible to obtain otherwise. Start by reading the numerous blogs written by individuals with disabilities. They are inspiringly, often times brutally, honest. Start watching the variety of YouTube videos individuals with disabilities have prepared for entertainment or education. There is a stand-up comedian with Cerebral Palsy named Josh Blue that is hysterical. I have yet to see the show of Kathy Buckley, a deaf comedian that has been delivering successful comedy routines for decades. I have heard she is fantastically funny.

Joining an organization that focuses on self-improvement, like Toastmasters, will put you in touch with many people with disabilities. It does not take long to discover that there is much more to an individual with a disability than what meets the eye. That "much more" is often an extraordinary gift or talent, an inspiring level of courage, a beyond-the-years wisdom, a great sense of humor, or a wellspring of compassion and unconditional love.

These qualities are extolled on some of the more famous disabled: Helen Keller, Stevie Wonder, Stephen Hawking, and the late Christopher Reeves. There are thousands upon thousands more, equally inspiring.

By becoming comfortable with and open to those with disabilities, we open ourselves to a treasure trove of surprises and delights sure to please us.

What Works for Me

The daughter of a lifelong friend made an interesting remark to me after reading my first book, *Read My Lips Tips for Success*. The book focuses on facing and overcoming adversity and I share the many challenges I have faced and have either overcome or learned to manage. One of those things is being very shy. "I never thought of you as shy, Linnaea!" she said.

I can easily explain that.

I do best in social situations as a "doer" rather than an "observer." That is, I like to be behind-the-scenes — someone that makes an event or party successful. By being a part of the "working crew", I have more control over what is happening around me. For example, at a party, serving as a super host, I don't need to stand and make conversation with people. Instead, I am flitting about making sure people are comfortable. "Would you like another drink?" or "Did you know there is a hot tub outside you can enjoy?" things like that. If a hearing situation gets awkward, I can excuse myself saying I am needed in the kitchen.

Earlier in this book, I mentioned I was videotaping at a conference. I do a lot of videotaping at events. Not only because I love doing it, but also because it, again, is a "behind-the-scenes" function. People usually don't talk to me much as I'm doing an important job. I can participate in a very significant way without ignoring anyone. I can have fun.

So, for me, if someone asks me to an event, or asks me to help out at an event, the first thing I'll ask is" How can I help?" Putting me at a registration table, of course, doesn't work for me. It is a position that requires hearing accurately. The jobs that work best for me are those that have me in a "gopher" position. I don't feel inferior or intimidated in the least. I feel empowered to participate, to connect, all the while feeling safe.

This approach to handling my disability has worked well for me. I have survived and have enjoyed quite a few successes. The following observation from my brother Steve Lewis about my disability, my life, and me underscores the wisdom of Marlee Matlin's quote that opens this chapter:

"It was natural to worry when a childhood illness robbed my little sister of a significant portion of her hearing. Would she be able to cope with what seemed to be a crushing disability? What would her life be like? Just fine, as it has turned out!

Linnaea's ever-growing list of personal and professional accomplishments has led me to question the relevance of a "disability" with respect to a meaningful, successful, happy life. I have watched with awe and admiration as Linnaea has achieved success upon success in her professional life as a leader in developing distance-learning materials and programs at UCLA; has risen to the highest levels of public speaking in the Toastmasters organization; has written and delivered sermons that touch congregations at the deepest levels; has helped people celebrate and commemorate the lives of family and friends at services marking moments of transition.

I believe Linnaea's early "disability" has led to a life filled with compassionate understanding and empathy for others along with a burning desire to achieve whatever goals she sets her sights on. There was no need to worry."

I believe that if you are reading this book, you are opening the door for understanding and acceptance of another with a hearing loss — even if that other is yourself.

Chapter 17 References and Resources:

Kathie Snow site Disability is Natural:
http://www.disabilityisnatural.com/

Linnaea's book: Read My Lips Tips for Success:
http://www.linnaeamallette.com/books-by-linnaea-mallette/

Toastmasters International: http://Toastmasters.org

Josh Blue: http://joshblue.com/

ABOUT THE AUTHOR

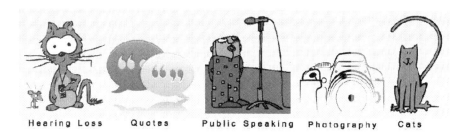

Hearing Loss   Quotes   Public Speaking   Photography   Cats

Linnaea Mallette is a professional speaker, trainer and author with five passions: Hearing Loss, Quotes, Public Speaking, Photography, and Cats.

Linnaea educates in an entertaining fashion about hearing loss — for those who have it and those who do not — through many speaking venues. The Hearing Loss Tips blog is at http://HearingLossTips.com.

Linnaea shares her experience and knowledge about mastering public speaking at http://KissSpeakingTips.com. She believes, based on her own experience, that mastering that #1 fear increases one's confidence and people achieve personal and professional success.

On Linnaea's blog she often shares insights that enabled her to overcome adversity, including her physical disability — a profound hearing loss. Linnaea authored a book by the same title which is being updated with new content and retitled "Tips to Get Out Of The Pits," due to be published early 2015. For 18 months, Linnaea hosted her own radio show — interviewing guests from all walks of life who have faced and overcome some sort of adversity. Her guests' challenges included child abuse, dyslexia, suicide, depression, preventing identity theft, overcoming fear of public speaking, grief, Parkinson's disease, and SO much more. Look for those podcasts on her personal webpage, LinnaeaMallette.com.

One of the hallmarks of the blog on Linnaea's website are the daily words of wisdom picture quotes designed to encourage and inspire. You can view the e-books she has created. They are free and accessible on the site. The blog is on http://linnaeamallette.com.

An offshoot of the words of wisdom work is Linnaea's newest revitalized passion, photography. Her photographs are available for royalty-free purchase at three stock photography sites:

Dreamstime: http://www.dreamstime.com/linnaeacat_info

PublicDomainPictures.net: http://bit.ly/lmonpdp

FOAP: https://www.foap.com/community/profiles/delightfuldistract ions

Linnaea also loves cats. As her book instructs, finding what brings you joy and focusing on it is critical to creating a life you love to live. To that end, she employs her talents in creating cat images and videos, and teaches others how to do the same at http://catwows.com

Linnaea is a Distinguished Past District Governor, Distinguished Toastmaster, and a Qualified Speaker for District 52, Toastmasters International. View her profile at http://www.linnaeamallette.com/speaking-and-training-with-linnaea-mallette.

Linnaea retired from a 33-year career at UCLA where in the last 12 years she was the Training Coordinator in Office of Research Administration. While in this position, she was featured in UCLA TODAY in 2002 (http://www.spotlight.ucla.edu/staff/linn_mallette/) and nominated for the Chancellor's "True Bruin" Award in 2012.

In 2002, she received the Oticon "Focus on People Award" for being one of 12 individuals nationwide to defy the stereotype of being hearing impaired.

Linnaea resides in the Greater Los Angeles area with her husband of 20 years and their beloved cat, Wilson Bones Mallette.

To contact Linnaea to speak at your organization or event, she can be reached (via email!) at lm@linnaeamallette.com or via her Hamilton CapTel number: 747-202-5698 OR Leave a message at Google Voice® 818-275-0632. Remember, email is best when reaching out to Linnaea.

Made in the USA
Lexington, KY
23 April 2015